TUMOURS OF LARYNX
A Clinicopathological Study

Dr Sangeeta Aggarwal

जय गुरुदेव

Full Color Plates
ISBN13: 978-93-92201-56-1 Paperback Edition
ISBN13: 978-93-92201-57-8 Hardbound Edition
ISBN13: 978-93-92201-58-5 Digital Edition
Black/White Plates
ISBN13: 978-93-92201-59-2 B/W Low Price Edition

Title: Tumours of Larynx
SubTitle: A Clinicopathological Study
Author: Dr Sangeeta Aggarwal

Printed and Published by
Devotees of Sri Sri Ravi Shankar Ashram
34 Sunny Enclave, Devigarh Road,
Patiala 147001, Punjab, India

https://advaita56.weebly.com/
The Art of Living Centre

https://www.artofliving.org/

1st Edition August 2012

Reprint with Notes November 2021

जय गुरुदेव

Dedication

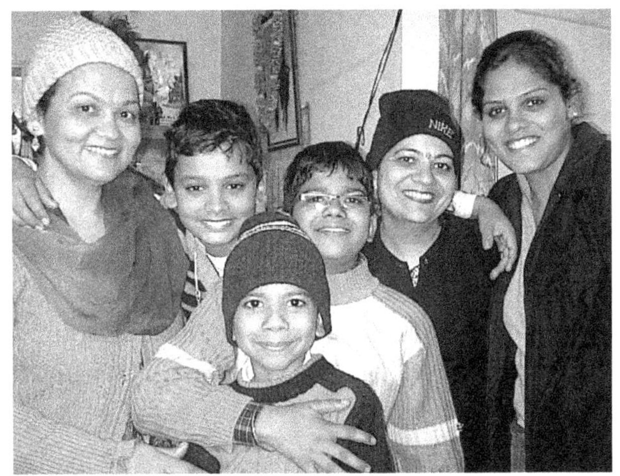

Dedicated to my Children & all the children Everywhere

Preface

This book 'Tumours of Larynx' is a work I have done during my post-graduation study. It has helped me to learn from the patients as I listened *carefully* and patiently. What they complain is a very *important* factor to be considered when making a diagnosis.

This disease incapacitates the patient for the whole life. The larynx protects the airway and if one cannot breathe one cannot survive, and if one has difficulty breathing, then each moment becomes unbearable. This disease which may be inferred by patient's history and diagnosed on *simple* clinical examination by laryngoscopy should be aware to medical students of every field. *No* expensive battery of tests is required to confirm the diagnosis.

Anatomy and physiology of larynx has been added in lucid detail so that its understanding becomes easier, and the book has been profusely illustrated with diagrams, working methods, reports, charts and tables.

I appreciate suggestions from readers and welcome their feedback.

Jai Gurudev.

Sangeeta Aggarwal
sangeeta_5339@yahoo.co.in
Sri Sri Global Meditating Doctors Association
https://www.artofliving.org/in-en/projects/rural-development/health/global-meditating-doctors-association

Foreword

My interactions with Dr Sangeeta Aggarwal date back the time when none of us knew each other by name, yet I was greatly impressed by the focus and dedication with which she used to volunteer for the Weekly Long Kriya – a one and a half hour combo of Yoga and Meditation drill . The clarity of her thoughts and precision of her action is amply reflected in the book you are holding in your hands right now. Being author of a book on Bio-medical Instrumentation, I understand the challenges one faces to convey subject matter to readers without any vagueness or loss of continuity. This book on Tumours of Larynx is reader-friendly, wherein the theme flows along the path of natural learning. It is common knowledge that tumours can be benign or malignant. This manuscript details in this classification and specifies its incidence on the basis of age, sex, socioeconomic status, occupation to state a few. Predisposing factors like substance abuse, poor orodental hygiene and vocal strain are adequately discussed. Next time when I get excited while delivering lectures to my students, and strain my vocals, these findings will help me contain the pitch of my voice.

   I am confident the reader, whether a student, a researcher or practicing physician, will benefit a lot from this book.
Sat Sri Akal.

Dr Mandeep Singh
Ph.D. (Telecardiology)
THAPAR UNIVERSITY
Patiala, India
https://www.thapar.edu/

Acknowledgements

I wish to express my sincere appreciation towards my teachers and colleagues whom I worked with.

It gives me immense pleasure to acknowledge with veneration and a sense of gratitude **Dr. B.S. Sohal**, *Associate Professor, Department of ENT, Government Medical College & Rajindra Hospital, Patiala.*

Words do not suffice to express my profound thanks to **Dr. Manjit S. Bal**, *Professor and Head, Department of Pathology, GMC&H, Patiala.*

It was with the grace of **Sri Sri Ravi Shankar** *my beloved Guruji that I could complete my work on time. I express my deep sense of belongingness to my parents for their love, unfailing attention to my needs and ever inspiring attitude that helped me to achieve whatever I have accomplished today. I am thankful to my brother* **monty** *for his cooperation throughout the project.*

Sangeeta Aggarwal

Table of Contents

TABLE OF DIAGRAMS

TABLE OF CHARTS

ABBREVIATIONS

BP	Blood pressure
BT	Bleeding time
Ca in situ	Carcinoma in situ
CT	Clotting time
CR No	Case registration number
CVS	Cardiovascular system
DLC	Differential leucocyte count
DOA	Date of admission
DOD	Date of discharge
ENT	Ear, Nose, Throat
ESR	Erythrocyte sedimentation rate
Hb	Haemoglobin
H/o	History of
HPV	Human papilloma virus
JVP	Jugular venous pressure
pCO_2	Partial pressure of carbon dioxide
pO_2	Partial pressure of oxygen
SCC	Squamous cell carcinoma
TLC	Total leucocyte count
TNM	Tumour Node Metastasis
VC	Vocal cord

Prayer

योगेन चित्तस्य पदेन वाचां मलं शरीरस्य च वैद्यकेन ।

योऽपाकरोतं प्रवरं मुनीनां पतञ्जलिं प्राञ्जलिरानतोऽस्मि ॥

yogena cittasya padena vācāṃ malaṃ śarīrasya ca vaidyakena |

yo'pākarotaṃ pravaraṃ munīnāṃ patañjaliṃ prāñjalirānato'smi ||
My heart feels Oneness with the Master who teaches Asana for the
MIND, Grammar for the TONGUE, Ayurveda for the BODY.

Chapter 1. INTRODUCTION

Only vertebrates with their thoracoabdominal diaphragms are able to use their larynges as flutter valves; altering air flow from their respiratory bellows to produce sound.

The production of sound for communication of complex information is limited to the highest orders. Thus, only in humans is the larynx significantly altered for voice production.

We are in very fortunate times, as we are moving into an era of more trust love, compassion, service and care for one another. We have now started caring more for the planet. Jai Gurudev.

H H Sri Sri Ravi Shankar, Dialogues on the New Age, Rishimukh Feb2008, www.artofliving.org

'I solemnly pledge to consecrate my life to the service of humanity' *from* The Declaration of Geneva, a declaration of physicians' dedication to the humanitarian goals of medicine.

World Medical Association www.wma.net

adapted from the Hippocratic Oath, regarded as father of western medicine

The larynx serves three basic functions in humans. In order of functional priority they are

- Protective
- Respiratory and
- Phonatory (Sasaki and Isaacson, 1988).

The larynx serves to protect the lower airways, facilitates respiration and plays a key role in phonation. In humans the protective and respiratory functions are compromised in favour of its phonatory function. The protective function is entirely reflexive and involuntary, whereas the respiratory and phonatory functions are initiated voluntarily but regulated involuntarily (Sasaki, 2006).

A surgical division into supraglottis, glottis and subglottis has embryologic and anatomic co-relates and historically has had value in predicting the patterns of tumour invasion and tumour behaviour (Adams and Maisel, 1998).

Tumour-Like Lesions & Tumours of the Larynx

Laryngeal Granulomas are often sequelae of surgery. They arise in mucosal defects subjected to severe mechanical stress; and also after bronchoscopy or intubation. Intubation granulomas occur mainly in women and children. A contact ulcer may give rise to a contact granuloma. The lesion recurs frequently. Microscopically the richly vascular granulation tissue may be covered by a thin layer of squamous epithelium.

Vocal Cord Nodules are usually symmetric and occur between the anterior and middle third of each vocal cord, most frequently in children. These are less frequent in women than in men. In men they may reflect an occupational vocal strain e.g. teachers, army officers. Microscopically subepithelial edema is accompanied by nodular fibrosis of varied density and hyalinization.

Vocal Cord Polyps of the larynx are smooth, rounded, sessile or pedunculated nodules that rarely exceed 1cm in diameter and occur most often on the true vocal cords. They are frequently found in singers and sometimes designated as "singer's nodules". A vocal strain is often associated with vocal cord polyps. Three main structural variants occur, often within the same lesion: Edematous, highly vascular and fibrous polyps. Men of age between 30-50 years are affected twice as frequently as women. The anterior half of the vocal cords and the adjacent area of the anterior subglottis are the most common sites. Bilateral polyps occur in about 20%. Translucent pedunculated polyps vary in size from a few millimetres to 1 cm. The highly vascular type tends to be opaque and congested. The fibrous variant is firm, white and opalescent. Microscopically the surface of the edematous polyp is covered by thin squamous epithelium. The often myxoid stroma contains scant cells and consists mainly of an intercellular, poorly stained ground substance with some collagenous fibres. The vascular type displays a highly cellular stroma with collagenous fibres and numerous blood vessels. The telangiectatic or angiomatous type may resemble a cavernous hemangioma. Thrombosis and hyaline changes often occur. The fibrous type possesses a fibrous stroma with few cells and blood vessels (Arnold, 1987).

Benign Tumours

EPITHELIAL TUMOURS

The **papilloma** is a true neoplasm that grows as a soft, succulent raspberry-like friable excrescence or nodule, usually on the true vocal cords. These lesions occur at any age and although usually single in adults may be multiple in children. The multiple juvenile papillomas often regress at puberty; they are now known to be caused by human papilloma virus (HPV 11). This is the most frequent of the benign tumours of the larynx. There are two important variants of papilloma, the juvenile and the adult form (Rains and Ritchie, 1984).

Juvenile Papilloma occurs in the first years of life and usually disappears during puberty. Both sexes are equally affected. The lesion is often multiple and widely distributed over the mucosal surface of the larynx (papillomatosis). The cause of juvenile papilloma is unknown. Macroscopically juvenile papillomas are soft, finely lobulated and pale pink, measuring usually 2 to 5 mm in diameter. Characteristically they are mobile. This is an important diagnostic feature, since fixed tumours should arouse suspicion of malignancy. Microscopically keratinisation is absent and there is no atypia. Recurrent papilloma has similar features. **Adult Papilloma** is the most frequent benign laryngeal neoplasm in adult (about 90%) with a predilection for men. It appears as a well-defined opaque and warty solitary lesion, preferentially on the vocal cords, but also on the floor of the ventricle and in the supraglottic space. Chemical agents, especially tobacco smoke and mechanical stress are probable etiological factors. Microscopically there is always some, often intensive keratinisation present (Arnold 1987).

ECTODERMAL TUMOURS

Adenomas are rare benign tumours arising from seromucinous glands of larynx. Most of these occur in subglottic larynx. Symptoms may be few until the tumour obstructs breathing. This accounts for less than 3% of all benign tumours of the larynx. It occurs mainly in the ventricle of Morgagni and in the ventricular fold protruding from the intact mucosal surface. Microscopy shows a tumour composed of tubular and acinar structures made of columnar and goblet cells. Oncocytic (eosinophilic) papillary cystadenoma can be difficult to distinguish from glandular hyperplasia with oncocytic features (Arnold 1987). **Neurogenic tumours**: Neurilemmoma is a benign tumour arising from Schwann cells of axon sheath. It is usually a well encapsulated slowly growing tumour which can be fairly large. Paraganglioma mostly arise from supraglottic paraganglia and less frequently from the subglottic area (Robin & Olofsson, 1997).

MESODERMAL TUMOURS

Vascular neoplasms arise from blood or lymphatic vessels. The tumours arising solely from lymph vessels are extremely rare within the larynx. Combined lymphangiomas and haemangiomas may be present. **Chondroma** is a cartilaginous tumour of larynx first described by Travers. It tends to occur between 40 and 70 years of age and is more frequent in men than in women with a ratio of 4:1. Most of these (70%) originate in the cricoid cartilage and most often from posterior cricoid plate (Robin & Olofsson, 1997).

MYOGENIC TUMOURS

Leiomyomas have been reported in children but they occur more often in adults of all ages. They seem to be most common in the supraglottic region and are of pea to pigeon-egg size. They have been removed endoscopically or by external approach. **Rhabdomyomas** of the true adult type are extremely rare tumours of skeletal muscle in larynx. Most originate in the vocal cord region and appear as a polypoid mass but may extend above and below the cords. **Granular cell tumours** are considered to be mesenchymal in origin. They occur mostly on the true vocal cord. **Fibromas** are composed of fibrillar connective tissue. They are round, firm, smooth and sessile or pedunculated. **Lipomas** arise from adipose tissue, especially in the false cords. Many lipomas arise in hypopharynx and extend into the larynx (Robin & Olofsson, 1997).

Malignant Tumours of the Larynx

About 95% of laryngeal carcinomas are typical squamous cell tumours. Rarely adenocarcinomas are seen, presumably arising from mucous glands. The tumour usually develops directly on the vocal cords, but it may arise above or below the cords, on the epiglottis or aryepiglottis folds, or in the pyriform sinuses.

Those confined within the larynx proper are termed intrinsic, whereas those that arise or extend outside the larynx are called extrinsic. They begin as in situ lesions that appear as pearly grey wrinkled plaques on the mucosal surface, ultimately ulcerating and fungating (Kumar et al, 2004).

Aetiology

To most people, a cause implies a condition that is both necessary and sufficient to produce a pre-specified result. The most widely accepted risk factors or associations for laryngeal cancer are listed below:

- Smoking
- Excessive alcohol intake
- Age and sex (increasing age and male sex)
- Infection with human papilloma virus
- Diets rich in spicy foods and low in green leafy vegetables, vitamin A
- Chewing of betel leaf
- Transplantation (possible association)
- Exposure to sulphuric acid and radiation
- Laryngopharyngeal reflux (Domanowski, 2006).

Clinical

Although the particular tumour, the site and the patient's constitution play key roles in any given individual, laryngeal cancers as a whole can cause any of the following findings, alone or in combination:

- Dysphagia
- Hoarseness
- Aspiration
- Blood-tinged sputum
- Fatigue and weakness
- Cachexia

- Dyspnoea

- Pain

- Halitosis

- Actual expectoration of tissue

- Neck masses

- Otalgia (Domanowski, 2006).

Imaging Studies

Plain radiography of the neck and chest may be useful in planning surgery. If metastases are already present in the chest, the therapeutic decision tree changes entirely (Domanowski, 2006).

Diagnostic Procedures

Direct laryngoscopy provides a view better than that obtained with indirect laryngoscopy.

Suspension laryngoscopy provides an excellent view of the extent of the tumour and the overall condition of the airway mucosa.

Fine needle aspiration (FNA) of a neck mass may yield a positive result when the certainty of a malignant lymph node is not 100%.

Single, well-targeted biopsy reveals the nature (type and perhaps grade) of the tumour. Several biopsy procedures may be extremely useful in mapping the tumour to optimally plan surgery (Domanowski, 2006).

Histological Findings

The vast majority of laryngeal cancers are of the squamous cell carcinoma variety. Variations include standard squamous cell carcinoma (in situ or invasive, well, moderately or poorly differentiated), verrucous carcinoma, spindle cell carcinoma, basaloid-squamous cell carcinoma and papillary squamous cell carcinoma. Other types of carcinoma are neuroendocrine carcinoma, lymphoepitheliomatous carcinoma, adenocarcinoma and rare tumours like sarcomas, lymphomas and metastases. Laryngeal squamous cell carcinoma histologically is similar in many ways to squamous cell carcinoma found elsewhere in the body. It arises in stages from hyperplasia and dysplasia of various degrees. The pathologists classify the degree of atypicality as follows: well, moderately, or poorly differentiated or undifferentiated (Domanowski, 2006).

Other Carcinoma

Adenoid cystic carcinoma is the most common laryngeal minor salivary gland neoplasm and has the same histology as salivary gland tumours. May be associated with squamous cell carcinoma, particularly if supraglottic and either high grade or solid variants. **Adenocarcinoma:** Non-salivary gland types are rare in larynx. **Lymphoepithelioma-like carcinoma:** Often mixed with classic squamous cell carcinoma. **Mucoepidermoid carcinoma** is very rare, usually supraglottic.

Metastases are rare. Renal cell carcinoma and melanoma are among most common; laryngeal lesion may be initial presenting lesion. Also breast and lung metastases can occur. Thyroid carcinomas involve larynx by direct extension.

Neuroendocrine carcinoma: Difficult to distinguish paraganglioma, carcinoid and small cell carcinoma in small biopsies without stains. Neuroendocrine carcinomas are most common non-squamous carcinoma of larynx. Gross: polypoid lesions 2 mm to 4 cm, arising in submucosa. Micro: large polyhedral cells with hyperchromatic nuclei; also anaplastic cells, areas of necrosis and mitotic figures.

Well differentiated neuroendocrine carcinoma (carcinoid tumour) is rare; <20 cases described. Micro: nests and cords of relatively uniform cells with salt and pepper chromatin; may have oncocytic cells, clear cells, spindle cells. DD: paraganglioma, medullary carcinoma.

Moderately differentiated neuroendocrine carcinoma (atypical carcinoid) is the most common nonsquamous malignancy of larynx. Micro: usually nests or sheets of epithelioid cells with round/oval nuclei (often with peripheral palisading), stippled chromatin, occasional nucleoli, variable hyperchromasia.

Poorly differentiated neuroendocrine carcinoma includes small cell carcinoma which is an aggressive tumour with common cervical, nodal and distant metastases. Micro: sheets of small to medium sized cells with minimal cytoplasm, hyperchromatic nuclei with no prominent nucleoli; resembles lung tumour; may have foci of squamous or glandular differentiation. DD: basaloid squamous cell carcinoma, solid variant of adenoid cystic carcinoma (Pernick, 2006).

Other Malignancies

Angiosarcoma is often associated with local radiation therapy. Gross: polypoid mass of epiglottis. **Liposarcoma** is common in males aged 37-77 years. Gross: yellow polypoid masses, 2-6 cm. Micro: often well differentiated liposarcomas with atypical cells, scattered lipoblasts and infiltration. **Lymphoma** is usually supraglottic. Diffuse large B cell lymphoma is most common subtype. **Melanoma** is rare; <100 cases reported. Micro: pleomorphic polygonal epithelioid cells or spindle cells; often with cytoplasmic and nuclear melanin; abnormal mitotic figures; may have in situ melanoma. **Paraganglioma** shows malignant behaviour in 3-25%; 15% recur locally. Micro: cell nests (Zellballen) surrounded by sustentacular cells. DD: moderately differentiated neuroendocrine carcinomas.

Chondrosarcoma: 0.5% of primary laryngeal tumours. Gross: usually 3 cm or more, invasion into bone of ossified laryngeal cartilage. Micro: diagnostic fields often small; have atypical, neoplastic chondrocytes with loss of normal architecture and distribution; and invasion of bone; laryngeal cartilage usually has undergone endochondral ossification. Low grade chondrosarcoma shows slight increase in cellularity, mild atypia with binucleated chondrocytes within 1 lacuna; difficult to distinguish from chondroma. High grade chondrosarcoma is hypercellular with enlarged, binucleated and multinucleated atypical cells with variable tumour necrosis. Dedifferentiated chondrosarcoma is also called chondrosarcoma with additional malignant mesenchymal component. DD: vocal process of arytenoid cartilage (normal finding), chondroid metaplasia, chondroma (Pernick, 2006).

HISTOLOGICAL EXAMINATION

Currently it is normal to acquire a specimen (biopsy) of the tumour by direct laryngoscopy and this is usually carried out under general anaesthesia (or local anaesthesia) allowing a careful and thorough direct examination of the tumour, biopsy material should include an adequate amount of tissue both from ulcerated areas and elsewhere if practicable. The biopsy material is important on three grounds:

1. Definitive diagnosis of malignancy is required because even the most benign looking polyp or nodule has occasionally been found to be malignant. Conversely, some active looking keratoses may not be malignant.
2. Identification of the type of tumour: While squamous carcinoma is undoubtedly the most common, other rare forms of malignancy are found and need individual consideration.

3. Often neglected, the degree of differentiation may be significant (Robin & Olofsson, 1997).

Laryngeal lesions are diverse in their behaviour and prognosis and thus classification is particularly important. Attempts at classification were begun as long ago as 1876. Over a period of years (since 1954) the International Union against Cancer (UICC) has undertaken the task of establishing a classification of a number of cancers, the larynx being one of the first and now agreement has been reached generally with the American Joint Committee (AJC) and other similar bodies (UICC) about what may become a definite classification, at least for a decade. The basis of the UICC classification is anatomical (Robin and Olofsson, 1997).

Laryngeal cancer staging has been useful for studies of cancer management and as a dynamic and modified grade of lesion size and location. It allows institutional series to be compared, allowing recognition of differences among different management groups. TNM staging is useful for discussing individual tumours in a patient and is required by institutions managing cancer patients and maintaining a tumour registry. (Joint Commission on Accreditation of Health care Organizations [JCAHO] requirement) (Adams & Maisel, 1998).

Anatomical Sites and Subsites

1. Supraglottis

   Epilarynx (including marginal zone)

   a. Suprahyoid epiglottis (including the tip)

   b. Aryepiglottic fold

   c. Arytenoids

   Supraglottis excluding epilarynx

   d. Infrahyoid epiglottis

   e. Ventricular bands (false cords)

   f. Ventricular cavities

2. Glottis

   a. Vocal cords

   b. Anterior commissure

   c. Posterior commissure

3. Subglottis

4. Regional Lymph nodes (the cervical nodes) (Robin & Olofsson, 1997).

TNM Clinical Classification

T – Primary tumour

TX – Primary tumour cannot be assessed

TO – No evidence of primary tumour

Tis – Carcinoma in situ

Supraglottis

T1   Tumour limited to one subsite of supraglottis with normal vocal

cord mobility

T2   Tumour invades more than one subsite of supraglottis or glottis

with normal vocal cord mobility

T3   Tumour limited to larynx with vocal cord fixation and/or invades

post-cricoid area, medial wall of pyriform sinus or pre-epiglottic

tissues

T4   Tumour invades through thyroid cartilage and/or extends to other

tissues beyond the larynx, e.g. to oropharynx, to soft tissues of neck

Glottis

T1   Tumour limited to vocal cord(s) – may involve anterior or posterior

commissures – with normal mobility

T1a   Tumour limited to one vocal cord

T1b   Tumour involves both vocal cords

T2   Tumour extends to supraglottis and/or subglottis and/or with impaired vocal cord mobility

T3   Tumour limited to larynx with vocal cord fixation

T4   Tumour invades through thyroid cartilage and/or extends to other

tissues beyond the larynx.

Subglottis

T1   Tumour limited to the subglottis

T2   Tumour extends to vocal cord(s) with normal or impaired mobility

T3   Tumour limited to larynx with vocal cord fixation

T4   Tumour invades through cricoid or thyroid cartilage and/or

extends to other tissues beyond the larynx.

N   **Regional lymph nodes**

N1   Ipsilateral single ≤ 3 cm

N2   Ipsilateral single > 3 to 6 cm

        Ipsilateral multiple ≤ 6 cm

        Bilateral contralateral ≤ 6 cm

N3   > 6 cm

M   **Distant metastasis** (Robin & Olofsson, 1997).

Chapter 2. ANATOMICAL CONSIDERATIONS

The larynx is situated at the upper border of the trachea in the visceral compartment of the neck. It lies opposite the third to sixth cervical vertebra in adult males, being somewhat higher in women and children.

The average measurements of the larynx in adults are		
	Males	Females
Length	44 mm	36 mm
Transverse diameter	43 mm	41 mm
Sagittal diameter (antero-posterior)	36 mm	26 mm

(Standring, 2005).

SKELETON OF LARYNX

This is formed by a series of cartilages interconnected by ligaments and fibrous membranes and moved by a number of muscles (both intrinsic and extrinsic). It is lined by mucous membrane which is continuous above and behind with that of pharynx and below with that of trachea. The corniculate, cuneiform, tritiate and epiglottic cartilages and the apices of the arytenoid are composed of elastic fibrocartilage, with little tendency to calcify. The thyroid, cricoid and the greater part of the arytenoids cartilages consist of hyaline cartilage and may undergo mottled calcification as age advances, commencing about the twenty-fifth year in the thyroid cartilage and somewhat later in the cricoid and arytenoids. By the sixty-fifth year these cartilages commonly appear patchily dense in radiographs.

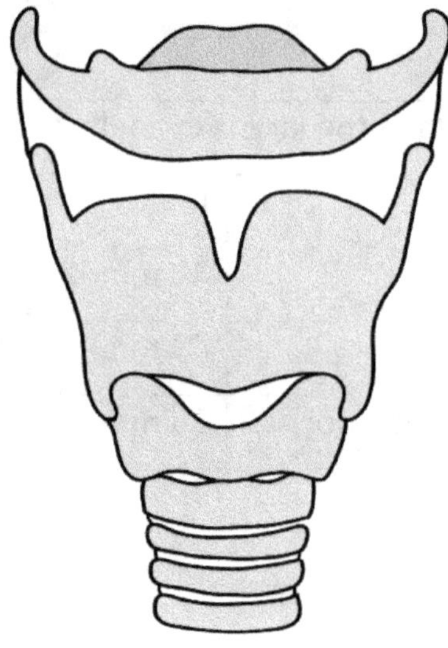

Fig(a) Unpaired Cartilages of Larynx

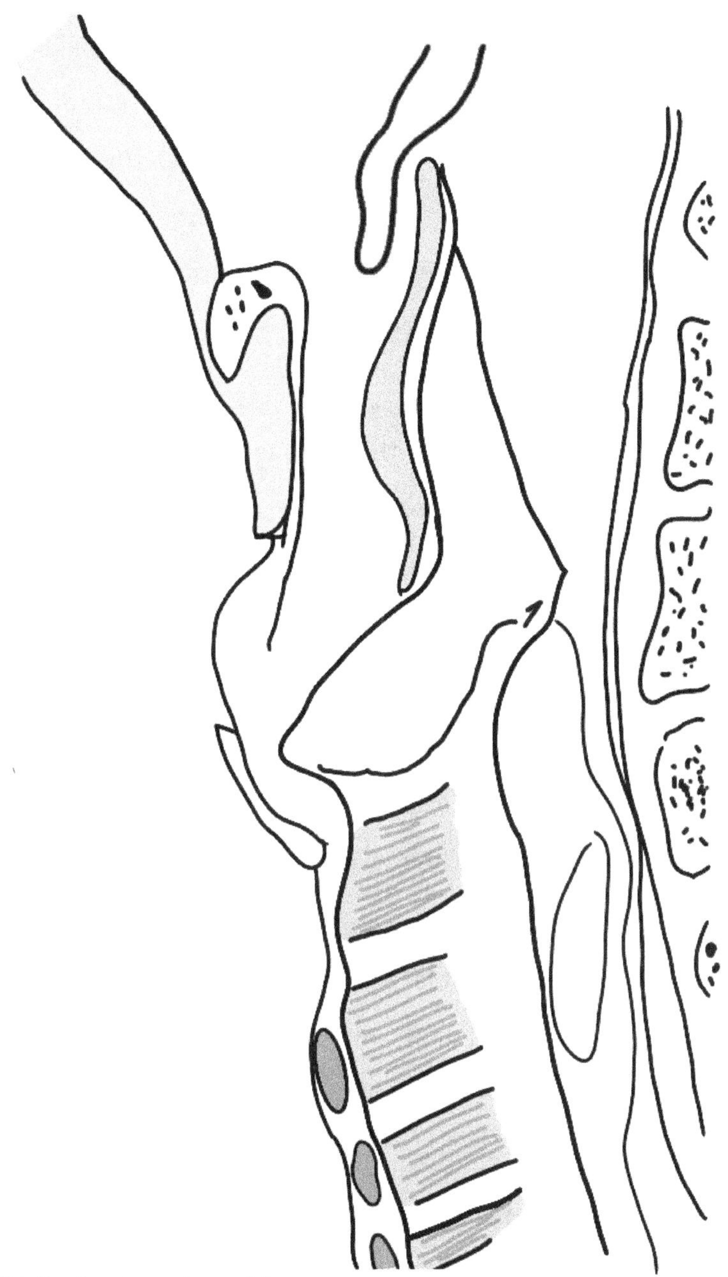

Fig(b) Sagittal section of Larynx

Epiglottis

is a thin leaf-like plate of elastic fibrocartilage, which projects obliquely upwards behind the tongue and hyoid body and in front of the laryngeal inlet. Its free end is broad and round. It is occasionally notched in the midline and is directed upwards. Its attached stalk is long and narrow and is connected by the elastic thyroepiglottic ligament to the back of the laryngeal prominence of the thyroid cartilage below the thyroid notch. Its sides are attached to the arytenoids cartilages by aryepiglottic folds.

Thyroid Cartilage is the largest of the laryngeal cartilages. It consists of two quadrilateral laminae whose anterior borders fuse along their inferior two-thirds at a median angle forming the subcutaneous laryngeal prominence – Adam's apple. Above, the laminae are separated by a V-shaped superior thyroid notch or incisure. Posteriorly the laminae diverge and their posterior borders are prolonged as slender horns, the superior and inferior cornua.

Cricoid Cartilage is attached below to the trachea and articulates with the thyroid cartilage and the two arytenoid cartilages by synovial joints. It forms a complete ring around the airway, the only laryngeal cartilage to do so. It is smaller but thicker and stronger than the thyroid cartilage. It has a narrow curved anterior arch and a broad flatter posterior lamina.

Arytenoid Cartilages are paired and articulate with the lateral parts of the superior border of the cricoid lamina. Each is pyramidal and has three surfaces, two processes, a base and an apex.

Corniculate Cartilages are two conical nodules of elastic fibrocartilage which articulate with the apices of the arytenoid cartilages prolonging them posteromedially. They lie in the posterior parts of the aryepiglottic mucosal folds and are sometimes fused with the arytenoid cartilages.

Cuneiform Cartilages are two small elongated club-like nodules of elastic fibrocartilage, one in each aryepiglottic fold anterosuperior to the corniculate cartilages. These are visible as whitish elevations through the mucosa.

Tritiate Cartilages are two small nodules of elastic cartilage situated one on either side above the larynx within the posterior free edge of the thyrohyoid membrane, about halfway between the superior cornu of the thyroid cartilage and the tip of the greater cornua of the hyoid bone.

JOINTS

Cricothyroid Joint lies between the inferior cornua of the thyroid cartilage and the sides of the cricoid cartilage and it is synovial. **Cricoarytenoid Joint** is a pair of synovial joint existing between the facets on the lateral parts of the upper border of the lamina of the cricoid cartilage and the bases of the arytenoids. **Arytenocorniculate Joint** is a synovial or cartilaginous joint linking the arytenoid and corniculate cartilages.

SOFT TISSUES

The skeletal framework of the larynx is interconnected by ligaments and fibrous membranes, of which the thyrohyoid, cricothyroid, quadrangular and cricovocal membranes are the most significant. The thyrohyoid membrane is external to the larynx, whereas the paired quadrangular and cricovocal membranes are internal. All the membranes are composed of fibroelastic tissue. The named ligaments are the median cricothyroid ligament, the hyoepiglottic and thyroepiglottic ligaments; and the cricotracheal ligament.

Extrinsic Ligaments and Membranes

Thyrohyoid membrane is a broad fibroelastic layer attached below to the superior border of the thyroid cartilage lamina and the front of its superior cornua; and above to the superior margin of the body and greater cornua of the hyoid. It thus ascends behind the concave posterior surface of the hyoid, separated from its body by a bursa which facilitates the ascent of the larynx during swallowing.

Hyo- and thyroepiglottic ligaments: The epiglottis is attached to the hyoid bone and thyroid cartilage by the extrinsic hyoepiglottic and intrinsic thyroepiglottic ligaments respectively.

Cricotracheal ligament unites the lower cricoid border to the first tracheal cartilage and is thus continuous with the perichondrium of the trachea.

Intrinsic Ligaments and Membranes

Quadrangular membrane passes from the lateral margin of the epiglottis to the arytenoid cartilage on its own side. It is often poorly defined.

Cricothyroid ligament and cricovocal membrane: The cricothyroid ligament is composed mainly of elastic tissue. It consists of two parts: the anterior cricothyroid ligament and the lateral cricovocal membrane. The cricothyroid membrane passes upwards from the upper border of the cricoid cartilage to the lower border of the thyroid cartilage. Anteriorly it is thickened to form the anterior cricothyroid ligament which is broader below and narrower above. The cricovocal membrane is thinner than the anterior cricothyroid ligament. It arises beneath the cricothyroid membrane from the inner surface of the cricoid cartilage near its lower margin.

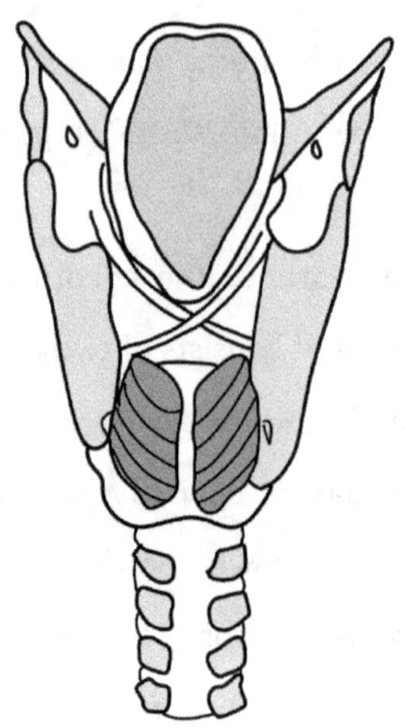
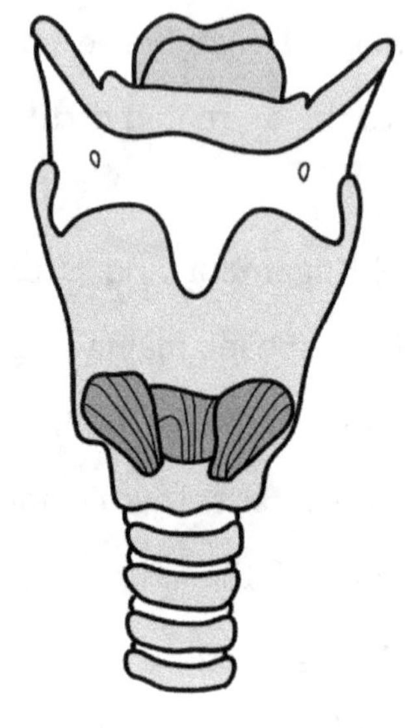

Fig(c) Larynx Posterior View   Anterior View

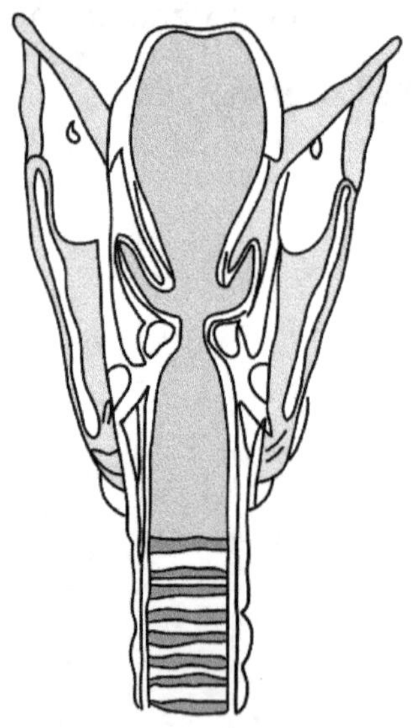
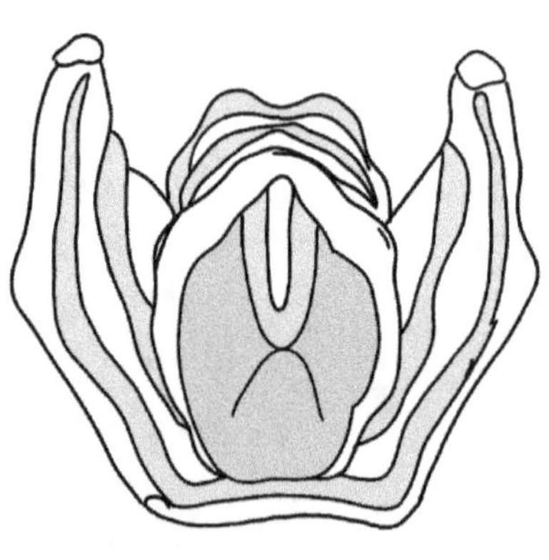

Larynx Coronal View   Top View

LARYNGEAL CAVITY

It extends from the laryngeal inlet down to the lower border of the cricoid cartilage where it continues down to the trachea.

Supraglottis refers to that part of the larynx which lies above the glottis. It includes the laryngeal ventricle, the vestibular folds, laryngeal surface of the epiglottis, arytenoid cartilages and the laryngeal aspects of the aryepiglottic folds. Laryngeal inlet or aditus is the aperture between the larynx and pharynx. Aryepiglottic fold contains ligamentous and muscular fibres. The ligamentous fibres represent the free upper border of the quadrangular membrane. Laryngeal introitus denotes the space between the laryngeal inlet and vestibular folds. It is wide above, narrow below and higher anteriorly than posteriorly.

Middle Part of the laryngeal cavity or glottis is the smallest and extends from the rima vestibule above to the rima glottidis below. On each side it contains the vestibular folds, the ventricle and the saccule of the larynx. The ventricule of the larynx opens into the saccule of the larynx, a pouch which ascends forwards from the ventricle beneath the vestibular fold and thyroid cartilage and occasionally reaches the upper border of the cartilage. It is conical and curves slightly backwards; 60-70 mucous glands, sited in the submucosa, open onto its luminal surface. The free thickened upper edge of the cricovocal membrane forms the vocal ligaments. It stretches back from either side from the midlevel of the thyroid angle to the vocal processes of the arytenoids. When covered by mucosa, it is termed the vocal cord. The vocal cords form the anterolateral edges of the rima glottidis and are concerned with sound production. Rima glottidis or glottis is the fissure between the vocal cords anteriorly and the arytenoid cartilages posteriorly. It is bounded behind by the mucosa passing between the arytenoid cartilages at the level of the vocal cords.

Subglottis is the lower part of the laryngeal cavity that extends from the vocal cords to the lower border of the cricoid.

THE PARALUMENAL SPACES

A number of potential spaces or compartments can be identified in and around the larynx. The three most commonly considered are the pre-epiglottic, the paraglottic and the subglottic spaces. They are not closed compartments and their existence does not preclude the spread of tumours.

The Pre-Epiglottic Space lies anterior to the epiglottis and also extends beyond the lateral margins of the epiglottis which gives it the form of a horse-shoe. It is primarily filled with adipose tissue and appears to contain no lymph nodes. The Paraglottic Space is a region of adipose tissue which contains the anterior laryngeal nerve, the laryngeal ventricle and part, or all, of the laryngeal saccule. It is bounded laterally by the thyroid cartilage and thyrohyoid membrane. Superomedially it is usually continuous with the pre-epiglottic space although it may be partitioned from it by a fibrous septum. The Subglottic Space is bounded laterally by the cricovocal membrane, medially by the mucosa of the subglottic region and above by the undersurface of Broyle's ligament in the midline. It is continuous below with the inner surface of the cricoid cartilage and its mucosa.

MUSCLES

Muscles of the larynx may be divided into extrinsic and intrinsic groups. The extrinsic muscles connect the larynx to neighbouring structures and are responsible for moving it vertically during phonation and swallowing. They include the infrahyoid strap muscles, i.e. thyrohyoid, sternothyroid and sternohyoid; and the inferior constrictor muscle of the pharynx. Two of the three elevator muscles of the pharynx, i.e. stylo- and palatopharyngeus, are also connected directly to the thyroid cartilage, mainly to the posterior aspect of the thyroid lamina and cornu.

Intrinsic Muscles: The oblique arytenoid lies superficial to the transverse arytenoid and is sometimes considered to be part of it. They cross each other obliquely at the back of the larynx, each extending from the back of the muscular process of one arytenoid cartilage to the apex of the opposite one. Some fibres continue laterally round the arytenoid apex into the aryepiglottic fold, forming the aryepiglottic muscle. **Transverse arytenoid** is a single unpaired muscle which bridges the gap at the back of the larynx between the two arytenoid cartilages and fills their posterior concave surfaces. It is attached to the back of the muscular process and adjacent lateral border of both arytenoids. **Posterior cricoarytenoid** arises from the posterior surface of the cricoid lamina. Its fibres ascend laterally and converge to insert on the back of the muscular process of the ipsilateral arytenoid cartilage. **Lateral cricoarytenoid** is attached anteriorly to the upper border of the cricoid arch. It ascends obliquely backwards to be attached to the front of the muscular process of the ipsilateral arytenoid cartilage. **Cricothyroid** is attached anteriorly to the external aspect of the arch of the cricoid cartilage. Its fibres pass backwards and diverge into two groups, a lower oblique part which slants backwards and laterally to the anterior border of the inferior cornu of the thyroid; and a superior straight part which ascends more steeply backwards to the posterior part of the lower border of the thyroid lamina.

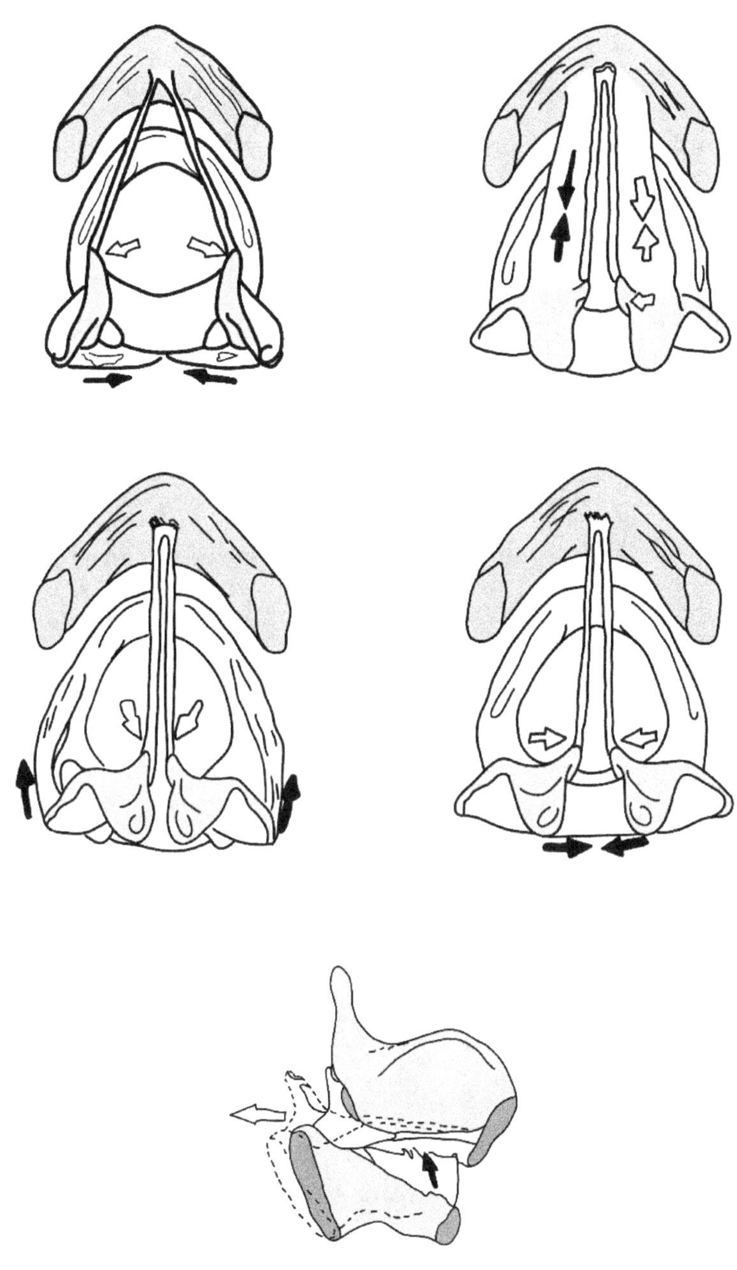

Fig(d) Muscles acting on Vocal cords

Thyroarytenoid and vocalis is a broad thin muscle lying lateral to the vocal cord, cricovocal membrane, laryngeal ventricle and saccule. It is attached anteriorly to the lower half of the angle of the thyroid cartilage and to the cricothyroid ligament. Its fibres pass backwards laterally and upwards to the anterolateral surface of the arytenoid cartilage. Its lower and deeper fibres form a band which in a coronal section appears as a triangular bundle. It is attached to the lateral surface of the vocal process and to the inferior impression on the anterolateral surface of the arytenoid cartilage. This bundle, the vocalis muscle, is parallel with and just lateral to the vocal ligament.

Thyroepiglotticus: Many of the fibres of the thyroarytenoid are prolonged into the aryepiglottic fold, where some terminate and others continue to the epiglottic margin as the thyroepiglottic muscle. The thyroepiglotticus can widen the inlet of the larynx by their action on the aryepiglottic folds.

THE INFANT LARYNX

This differs markedly form the adult larynx. Its cavity is short and funnel shaped. It is about one-third the size of the adult, although it is proportionately larger and this has two main consequences. First its lumen is disproportionately narrower than the adult and second, it lies higher in the neck than the adult larynx. At rest the upper border of the epiglottis is at the level of the second or third cervical vertebra and when the larynx is elevated it reaches the level of the first cervical vertebra. This high position is associated with the ability of the infant to use its nasal airway to breathe while suckling. The epiglottis is X-shaped with a furled petiole and the laryngeal cartilages are softer and more pliable than the adult larynx. The thyroid cartilage is shorter and broader than in the adult and lies closer to the hyoid bone in the neonate.

VASCULAR SUPPLY AND LYMPHATIC DRAINAGE

The blood supply of the larynx is derived mainly from the superior and inferior laryngeal arteries. Rich anastomoses exist between the corresponding contralateral laryngeal arteries and between the ipsilateral laryngeal arteries.

Superior Laryngeal Artery is normally derived from the superior thyroid artery, a branch of the external carotid artery, as this artery passes down towards the upper pole of thyroid gland. It runs down towards the larynx with the internal branch of the superior laryngeal nerve lying above it. It enters the larynx by penetrating the thyrohyoid membrane and divides into a number of branches which supply the larynx from the tip of the epiglottis down to the inferior margin of thyroarytenoid.

Inferior Laryngeal Artery is smaller than the superior laryngeal artery. It is a branch of the inferior thyroid artery which arises from the thyrocervical trunk of the subclavian artery. It ascends on the trachea with the recurrent laryngeal nerve, enters the larynx at the lower border of the inferior constrictor, just behind the cricothyroid articulation and supplies the laryngeal muscles and mucosa. It anastomoses with its contralateral fellow and with the superior laryngeal branch of the superior thyroid artery.

Superior and inferior laryngeal veins: Venous return from the larynx occurs via superior and inferior laryngeal veins which run parallel to the laryngeal arteries. They are tributaries of the superior and inferior thyroid veins respectively. The superior thyroid vein drains into the internal jugular vein and the inferior thyroid vein usually into the left brachiocephalic vein.

Lymphatic Drainage: The lymph vessels draining the supraglottic part of the larynx above the vocal cords accompany the superior laryngeal artery, pierce the thyrohyoid membrane and end in the upper deep cervical lymph nodes, often bilaterally. The supraglottic lymphatics also communicate with those at the base of the tongue. The vocal cords with their firmly bound mucosa and paucity of lymphatics provide a clear demarcation between the upper and lower areas of the larynx. Below the vocal cords, some of the lymph vessels pass through the cricovocal membrane to reach the prelaryngeal and/or pretracheal lymph nodes. Others run with the inferior laryngeal artery to join the lower deep cervical nodes.

INNERVATION

The larynx is innervated by the internal and external branches of the superior laryngeal nerve, the recurrent laryngeal nerve and sympathetic nerves. The internal laryngeal nerve is sensory, the external laryngeal nerve is motor and the recurrent laryngeal nerve is mixed. All the intrinsic muscles of the larynx are supplied by the recurrent laryngeal nerve except for cricothyroid, which is supplied by the external laryngeal nerve.

Superior laryngeal nerve arises from the middle of the inferior ganglion. The superior laryngeal nerve divides into two branches, a smaller external and a larger internal branch 1.5 cm below the ganglion.

Internal laryngeal nerve passes forwards 7 mm before piercing the thyrohyoid membrane, usually at a higher level than the superior thyroid artery. It splits into superior, middle and inferior branches on entering the larynx. The superior branch supplies the mucosa of the pyriform fossa. The large middle branch is distributed to the mucosa of the ventricle, specifically the quadrangular membrane. The inferior ramus is mainly distributed to the mucosa of the ventricle and subglottic cavity.

External laryngeal nerve passes beneath the attachment of sternothyroid to the oblique line of the thyroid cartilage and supplies cricothyroid.

Recurrent Laryngeal nerve: The upper part of this nerve has a close but variable relationship to the inferior thyroid artery. The nerve enters the larynx by passing deep to the fibres of cricopharyngeus and supplies this muscle. At this point the nerve is in intimate proximity to the posteromedial aspect of the thyroid gland. The main trunk divides into two or more branches usually below the lower border of the inferior constrictor. The anterior branch is mainly motor and the posterior branch is mainly sensory. The first ramus of the main motor branch of the recurrent laryngeal nerve innervates posterior cricoarytenoid, interarytenoid and lateral cricoarytenoid, before it terminates in thyroarytenoid. The right recurrent laryngeal nerve arises directly from the vagus nerve trunk high up in the neck and enters the larynx close to the inferior pole of the thyroid gland.

Autonomic supply to the larynx: Parasympathetic, secretomotor fibres run with both the superior and recurrent laryngeal nerves to mucous glands throughout the larynx. Postganglionic sympathetic fibres run into the larynx with its blood supply and have their origin in the superior and middle cervical ganglia (Standring, 2005).

Chapter 3. PHYSIOLOGY OF LARYNX

The larynx serves to protect the lower airways, facilitates respiration and plays a key role in phonation. In humans the protective and respiratory functions are compromised in favor of its phonatory function.

The protective function is entirely reflexive and involuntary, whereas the respiratory and phonatory functions are initiated voluntarily but regulated involuntarily.

Water-aerosol inhalation stimulation in partial upper airway obstruction activates water chemoreceptors on the epiglottis and causes reflex respiratory slowing and increase in tidal volume.

Abduction of the vocal cords during respiration is brought about by the posterior cricoarytenoid muscle, whereas their adduction involves all the intrinsic muscles, particularly the thyroarytenoid and cricoarytenoid muscles.

Reflexive glottic closure is achieved by simultaneous adduction of both vocal cords. Anesthesia and sedation impair reflexive vocal cord closure and predispose to aspiration.

Reflexive glottic closure is inhibited by hypothermia, inspiratory phase, increased arterial pCO_2, decreased arterial pO_2 and positive intrathoracic pressure. It is facilitated by hyperthermia, expiratory phase, decreased pCO_2, increased pO_2 and negative intrathoracic pressure.

Laryngeal denervation leads to vocal dysfunction and aspiration during swallowing.

Tracheostomy itself leads to centrally mediated impaired reflexes and decannulation (adductor failure and vocal cord fusion).

False vocal cords, even if denervated, resist air flow from the lower respiratory tract and serve expectorative function. The true vocal cords resist air flow from outside and play a protective role in respiration, thus explaining the difficulty in overcoming laryngospasm by abrupt pressure peaks from above (Sasaki, 2006).

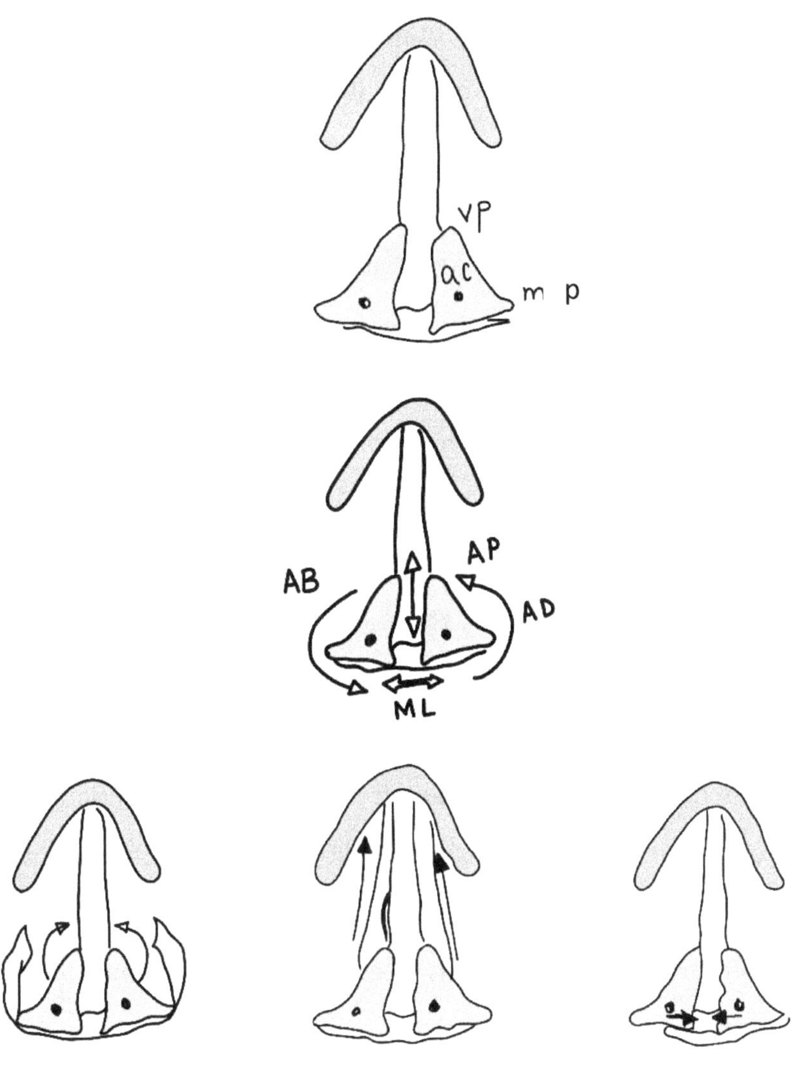

Fig(e) Movements of Vocal cord

STRUCTURE AND FUNCTION

The upper airway in adult humans traverses the digestive tract in the region of the pharynx, complicating its sphincteric protection of the lower airway. By sharing a common passageway with the upper digestive system, the larynx is also compromised in its respiratory performance by resultant ventilatory turbulence and, therefore, resistance. Thus, the anatomic configuration in adult humans that benefits phonatory purposes of the larynx simultaneously serves to compromise its sphincteric and respiratory functions. This functional dilemma is resolved at the laryngopharyngeal level by two important organic modifications: structural adaptation and delicate coordination among the three basic laryngeal functions as determined by precisely organized brainstem reflexes.

In adult humans the characteristic flat, shield-like configuration of the epiglottis serves to direct swallowed food laterally into the pyriform fossae, away from the midline laryngeal aperture. Furthermore, in adult humans, elevation of the larynx toward the nasal cavity during the height of deglutition exaggerates this protective function. Implicit in this manoeuvre is the role of the aryepiglottic folds, which consist of mucous membrane, connective tissue and muscle, extending from the epiglottic framework to the arytenoid bodies posteriorly. These lateral folds act as ramparts to the larynx, allowing food to pass on either side of the epiglottis along the gutter produced between each fold and the lateral pharyngeal wall. In this capacity, the cartilages of Santorini and Wrisberg, also called corniculate and cuneiform cartilages, respectively, are contained in the aryepiglottic folds to provide added support and stiffness to these ramparts of the laryngeal aperture. Therefore, from a structural perspective alone, it would appear that the primary role of the supraglottic larynx in adult humans lies in its protection of the lower airway.

In the human larynx the ability to perform as an effective valve depends on the unique shelf-like configuration of its superior and inferior folds bilaterally represented. The ventricular folds or false cords, which are located superiorly, act as exit valves, preventing the escape of air from the lower respiratory tract. When positioned by muscular contraction, they seal even more tightly as tracheal pressure is increased from below. This feature of adducted false cords occurs independently of muscle tone, a phenomenon attributable to their unique shape, which is characterized by the down-turned direction of their free margins. Such a configuration is made possible by the lateral ventricles and is exaggerated by the superior extension of the laryngeal saccules.

The false cords prevent the egress of air from the lungs and the true cords with their up-turned margins are capable of impeding its ingress; these views were confirmed by Lindsay on tomographic analysis of the larynx. Therefore, it is not surprising that expectorative functions of the larynx remain unimpaired in bilateral laryngeal paralysis. In this regard, passive closure of the false cords alone appears essential to effective cough production. The valvular component of the true cords, on the other hand, is implicated in the clinical difficulty experienced in overcoming laryngeal spasm by abrupt pressure peaks of positive pressure ventilation that only further serve to protectively seal the true cords. Therefore, from a structural perspective the false cords provide an expectorative function, whereas the true cords assume a protective role in respiration.

In humans, one must appreciate that both protective and respiratory functions of the larynx have been compromised in favor of its phonatory purposes. This unique compromise is reflected in part by compensatory structural modifications discussed above.

Basic functions of the larynx (protective, respiratory and phonatory) are derived from a complex interrelationship of diverse polysynaptic brainstem reflexes. On the one hand, protective function is entirely reflexive and involuntary, constituting one end of a spectrum that is balanced on the other by respiratory and phonatory performances that may be initiated voluntarily but regulated involuntarily through an array of feedback reflexes.

NEUROPHYSIOLOGY OF PHONATION

The phonatory function of the larynx is probably the least well understood of its three basic functions.

It is generally agreed that speech results from the production of a fundamental tone produced at the larynx and is modified by resonating chambers of the upper aerodigestive tract. Intelligible speech, therefore, represents the combined effect of the larynx, tongue, palate and related structures of the oral vestibule. The production of the fundamental tone is due to the vibration of the vocal folds against each other, generated by the passage of air between them. Vocal cord vibrations may be a passive phenomenon representing the basis of the aerodynamic theory of sound generation. Such a theory finds support in the observation that the completely paralyzed larynx is capable of producing sound, as is the cadaver larynx when subglottic pressure is forcefully increased. Obviously, phonation ceases when a tracheotomy is performed for diversionary purposes.

Although sound production may be considered a passive function, the regulation of its acoustic quality is not a passive phenomenon. Rather, vocal cord shaping and positioning are under active neural regulation.

The cricothyroid muscle increases fundamental frequency (F0) by tensing the vocal fold. The vocal fold is stretched, elongated, thinned and slightly adducted to the paramedian position as the vocal fold is lowered within the larynx. These changes reduce the cross-sectional area of the vocal fold, reducing vibratory mass and increasing F0. Vocalis muscle, on the other hand, generates the opposite effect as it loosens and thickens the vocal fold. In addition, as it increases glottal resistance, it contributes to vocal intensity as subglottal pressure is increased. Vocal control, therefore, is achieved by the coordinated efforts of respiratory, laryngeal and articulatory muscles capable of producing great variations of tonal qualities characterizing the human voice (Sasaki, 2006).

Chapter 4. REVIEW OF LITERATURE

FREQUENCY

The ratio of benign to malignant tumours of the larynx is about 1:10. Most frequent types of benign tumours are papillomas (juvenile and adult papillomas). Adenomas account for less than 3% of all benign tumours of the larynx (Arnold et al, 1987).

Head and Neck cancers constitute a major health problem in India accounting for 23% of all cancers in males and 6% in females (ICMR, 1992). Out of these, cancer of the larynx constitutes 20% of the cases (Ahluwalia et al, 2001).

In India there are 25,000 new cases of Cancer Larynx every year (Simon, 2005). Carcinoma of larynx is a common disease in North Indian population, commonly seen in smokers and alcoholics and poses a serious health problem (Bakshi, 2004). In Chennai, the highest incidence of cancer in the whole body is in the region of head and neck. Out of which, larynx is the commonest site of cancer. It is one among the few cancers having a very good prognosis. It is because early diagnosis is possible and excellent treatment modalities and rehabilitation advancements are available. Cancer larynx is more common in men than in women (8: 1 ratio) and is usually seen over 50 (Simon, 2005).

India has a population of more than 1 billion, of whom 3 million will have cancer at any one time, with an annual incidence of approximately 1 million new patients. While cancer is not a common disease in India, an increasing elderly population ensures that the number of people with cancer will increase in the future. It is difficult to obtain accurate cancer statistics in a large country such as India where only 6 cancer registries function for a population of 1 billion. However, the population based cancer registry in Mumbai (Bombay) has provided the age adjusted incidence rates of the 10 leading cancers for men and women (Smith, 2003).

Table: Age-standardized incidence rates* for 10 leading cancer sites in India

Men		Women	
Site	**Rate per 100,000**	**Site**	**Rate per 100,000**
Lung	10.7	Breast	28.1
Oesophagus	7.3	Cervix	17.1
Prostate	6.8	Ovary	8.2
Larynx	6.2	Oesophagus	6.2
Stomach	5.5	Lung	4.5
Tongue	5.5	Leukaemia	3.6
Lymphomas	4.8	Stomach	3.5
Hypopharynx	4.5	Uterus	3.4
Liver	4.4	Lymphoma	3.4
Leukaemia	4.3	Colon	2.7

* Adjusted to the world population, aged between 0 and 74 years, as suggested by the World Health Organization (Smith, 2003).

Holinger et al (1968) mentioned that laryngeal papilloma was more common in adults. Of the 174 patients with laryngeal papilloma in the past 15 years, 74 were under 13 years of age and 97 were 13 years of age or more. Males were 38 as compared to 39 females in the first group and 64 males as compared to 33 females in the second group. This indicates equal sex distribution in pre-puberty age and predominance of males in post-puberty.

Rowley and Boles (1972) in a review of ten years record of 118 supraglottic laryngeal carcinomas, found that 74% of the patients were in their 6th to 7th decade. Out of these 70% were heavy smokers, 7% were moderate and light smokers.

Stell and McGill (1975) in a study of 119 laryngeal cancers showed the significance of exposure to asbestos dust. 27.7% of the total patients had significant exposure to asbestos dust. Maximum age of onset of carcinoma was a decade less when compared with those of laryngeal carcinoma who had no history of exposure to asbestos.

Shaw (1979) cited that Friedmann had given statistics of benign tumours of larynx seen at the Institute of Laryngology and Otology, London, over a period of 21 years (1948-1969). He mentioned that 1122 cases were non-neoplastic. These included 72 retention cysts, 44 tubercular granulomas, 18 intubation granulomas, 14 contact ulcer granulomas, 13 amyloid deposits, 8 Wegener's granulomas, 6 granular cell myoblastomas and 3 were miscellaneous. These constituted 86% of total benign growths. Out of the remaining neoplastic benign tumours 170 were papillomas, 16 adenomas, 3 chondromas and 16 miscellaneous, which included fibroma, haemangioma, lipoma and neurofibroma. These constituted only 14% of the total growths. Thus non-neoplastic benign growths were more common.

Thomas (1979) conducted a survey at the Royal National Throat, Nose and Ear Hospital. 708 cases of carcinoma larynx were seen in 10 years from 1968 to 1977. The incidence was slightly less than 2% of all malignancies seen in this hospital. 700 cases were of squamous cell carcinoma, 1 of malignant melanoma of vocal cords, 2 chemodectomas, 1 chondrosarcoma, 1 plasmacytoma and 1 histiocytosis.

Arnold et al (1987) stated that the ratio of benign to malignant tumours of the larynx is about 1:10. Most frequent types of benign tumours are papillomas (juvenile and adult papillomas). Adenomas account for less than 3% of all benign tumours of the larynx.

Welkoborsky et al (1988) cited that neuroendrocrine tumours of the larynx are extremely rare. Only 20 cases of laryngeal carcinoid tumours have been reported. Since histological diagnosis is difficult, this unusual neoplasm was often misdiagnosed as an undifferentiated carcinoma.

Dinsdale et al (1990) reported a case of a 13 year old girl who presented with altered speech and dyspnoea on exertion for past 3 months. Physical examination revealed a pale yellow mass, 3 cm in diameter, pedunculated on the left aryepiglottic fold. Excisional biopsy of the mass was done and histopathology suggested a diagnosis of a typical myxoid lipogenic tumour. Only 70 cases of lipomatous laryngeal neoplasms have been reported in literature. They occur more frequently in men than in women (5:2) and have a peak incidence in the seventh decade. Typically, these grow slowly and cause dysphagia and voice changes without odynophagia.

Wilkinson III et al (1991) cited that laryngeal cartilaginous tumours classically arise from the cricoid or thyroid cartilage and are described as a tumour of the elderly population; with most occurring in persons over 50 years of age. They reported an unusual case of extraskeletal myxoid chondrosarcoma of the epiglottis in a young boy 15 years old.

Parker (1993) stated that sarcomas of the larynx are rare. Of all cancers, 2% are located in the larynx and less than 1% are of sarcomatous or mesenchymal origin. Chondrosarcoma is the most common of these sarcomas and differs from other sarcomas with respect to its origin and length of survival free of disease. 75% of these tumours originate in cricoid with 15% to 20% in thyroid cartilage.

According to Sharma et al (1995) neurilemmomas are neurogenic tumours arising from schwann sheath of peripheral, cranial, or sympathetic nerves. They reported a rare case of neurilemmoma arising from laryngeal surface of epiglottis and adjoining epiglottic fold. Most of the neurilemmomas are situated in supraglottic structures arising from branches of superior laryngeal nerve, the aryepiglottic fold being the commonest site. The nerve functions remain intact except in very large tumours because usually with the expansion of the tumour, the nerve fibre gets splayed over the capsule rather than becoming incorporated within the tumours.

Wenig and Heffner (1995) studied laryngeal and hypopharyngeal liposarcomas in seven men and one woman, in the age group 25 to 81 years. Symptoms included dysphagia, airway obstruction and the sensation of a foreign body in the throat. Histologically, seven of the tumours were of the biologically favourable types, representing either well-differentiated lipoma-like liposarcomas or myxoid liposarcomas. One tumour was a pleomorphic liposarcoma. Six of the eight patients had one or more episodes of recurrent tumour.

Wenig (1995) reported two cases of necrotizing sialometaplasia of the larynx. One case occurred in the subglottic larynx of a 37 year old woman and the other in the right false vocal cord of a 59 year old man. Excisional biopsy specimens showed fibrosis. Biopsy of the mass was diagnostic for a poorly differentiated squamous cell carcinoma with separate foci of necrotizing sialometaplasia.

Wenig (1995) showed that lipomas of the larynx are uncommon mesenchymal neoplasms. Two of the cases occurred in females and one in a male. Two cases involved the supraglottic larynx, the third involved the pyriform sinus. Symptoms included airway obstruction, dysphagia, throat discomfort and a sensation of excessive secretions in the throat. Clinically, a polypoid lesion described as yellow in appearance was seen.

According to Maurizi et al (1996) laryngeal verrucous squamous cell carcinoma (VSCC) of the larynx is a rare highly differentiated variant of squamous cell carcinoma and has specific morphological features and clinical behaviour. This tumour appears to be clinically malignant and histologically benign.

According to Barnes et al (1997) laryngeal paraganglioma originates in the neural crest cells in the laryngeal paraganglia. Two distinct types may be cited on the basis of clinical features, but biopsy is essential for diagnosis. By light microscopy, the Zellballen pattern appears pathognomonic.

Shirley (1997) cited that chondrosarcoma comprises 0.5% of all laryngeal tumours and only 0.1% of all head and neck malignancies. Approximately 200 cases of chondroma and chondrosarcoma of the larynx have been reported in the literature. Males predominate at a ratio of 3:1. The cases are seven times as common in Caucasians as compared to African Americans.

Berge et al (1998) described osteosarcoma of larynx which is rarest of all malignant mesenchymal tumours of larynx. Its diagnosis is made by identification of osseous matrix i.e. osteoid and/or bone, produced by the malignant cells. Prognosis is usually poor with tendency for local-soft-tissue recurrence and early loco-regional and distant metastasis.

Cocks et al (1999) presented a case of 49 year old man with a 9 month history of hoarseness at presentation. He had smoked 40 cigarettes per day and drunk 60 to 70 units of alcohol per week all his adult life. Indirect laryngoscopy revealed a lesion on the right vocal cord with possible subglottic extension and no palpable lymph nodes. Direct laryngoscopy and biopsy of lesion confirmed the histology to be leiomyosarcoma.

Sood et al (1999) documented two cases of carcinoid tumour of the larynx. Primary neuroendrocrine cases of the larynx are rare (accounting for 0.6% of laryngeal tumours) and are pathologically divided into three groups: (1) Carcinoid tumours which reportedly account for only 3% of neuroendrocrine lesions in this site (2) Atypical carcinoid tumours and (3) Small cell carcinomas.

According to Thompson et al (1999) exophytic and papillary squamous cell carcinomas (SCCs) are uncommon variants of SCC of the upper aero-digestive tract mucosa. 104 cases were identified which included 25 women and 79 men aged 27 to 89 years. Patients had hoarseness of voice at presentation and most patients were using tobacco (87) and/or alcohol (49).

According to Esposito et al (2001) occult cervical lymph node metastasis may often be associated with cancers of supraglottic larynx. In their series the incidence of occult lymph node metastases was 27%.   So there is general agreement in the literature that surgical treatment of the primary tumour should be performed in conjunction with bilateral neck dissection.

Lin et al (2001) reported a case of an Asian woman of primary melanoma of larynx. She had a polypoid tumour and four flat patches over the supraglottic region. Microscopically both "in situ change" and "melanosis" were noted. Mucosal malignant melanoma is an uncommon tumour of larynx and only 52 cases have been reported in literature mostly among white men.

According to Loos et al (2001) primary laryngeal angiosarcoma is rare. Five patients were studied. Three men and two women aged 29 to 71 years presented with hoarseness (4) and haemoptysis (1). Histologically, all tumours had anastomosing vascular channels lined by remarkably atypical endothelial cells protruding into the lumen, frequent atypical mitotic figures and haemorrhage.

Pham and Lannigan (2001) stated that carcinoma of larynx is a rare malignancy in the paediatric age group. A number of predisposing factors have been identified including juvenile laryngeal papillomatosis (JLP), radiation and tobacco exposure; and cancer malformation syndromes.

Wieneke et al (2001) showed that true giant cell tumours of the larynx are quite rare. Eight cases were studied – two women and six men, aged 26 to 62 years. Patients presented with a palpable neck mass (5 cases), airway obstruction (3 cases), hoarseness (3 cases) and dysphagia (2 cases). All tumours involved the thyroid cartilage, a few with local extension.

Fung et al (2002) studied primary larynx lymphomas, specifically of the mucosa-associated lymphoid tissue. They reported the first case in which both of these unusual findings were present, i.e. an extranodal marginal zone B-cell lymphoma of laryngeal mucosa-associated lymphoid tissue with Hodgkin-like transformation.

Hucumenoglu et al (2002) described a rare case of papillary adenocarcinoma arising from laryngeal surface of the epiglottis. It is a relatively slow growing and non-aggressive tumour. Glandular carcinomas of the larynx are rare tumours that constitute less than 1 % of all laryngeal malignancies.

Thompson and Gannon (2002) studied a total of 111 cases of chondrosarcoma of the larynx. These are rare tumours accounting for about 0.5% of all laryngeal primary tumours. There was a 3.6:1 male/female ratio of patients 25 to 91 years of age. Patients presented most frequently with hoarseness (72 cases). The majority of tumours involved the cricoid cartilage (77) with a mean size of 3.5 cm.

According to Thompson et al (2002) laryngeal spindle cell sarcomatoid carcinomas are uncommon tumours, frequently misdiagnosed as reactive lesions or mesenchymal malignancies. The records of 187 patients with tumours diagnosed as laryngeal spindle cell (sarcomatoid) carcinoma showed that there were 174 men and

13 women, 35 to 92 years of age (mean age 65.6 years). Nearly all patients experienced hoarseness of voice (88%), admitted to smoking (87%) and/or alcohol abuse (48%).

Khalil et al (2003) stated that paragangliomas of larynx are rare benign tumours that have to be differentiated from other neuroendocrine tumours. They reported that a recent review of English literature identified 65 cases. They are a subclass of neuroendocrine tumours with a neural origin. They showed a female to male preponderance of 3:1. Laryngeal paragangliomas are tumours of middle age with median age of 44 years.

Orlandi et al (2003) described a rare case of symptomatic nodular chondrometaplasia of laryngeal soft tissue. This has to be differentiated from true cartilaginous neoplasm of larynx such as chondroma and low grade chondrosarcoma.

Lee et al (2003) reported a case of adenoid cystic carcinoma (ACC) on the laryngeal surface of epiglottis mimicking a laryngeal cyst. ACC of the larynx is an infrequently encountered neoplasm that makes up less than 0.25% of all laryngeal carcinomas. The sites of origin in descending order are the subglottis, the supraglottis and the true glottis.

Sorrentino et al (2003) described angiosarcoma of the larynx which is a rare malignant tumour of vascular origin; accounting for less than 1% of all malignant tumours of the larynx. In some cases it is believed to be radiation induced. Angiosarcoma involves in particular the head and neck in areas such as scalp and face. They described a patient with hypopharyngolaryngeal angiosarcoma who presented with dysphagia, dysphonia and a palpable right latero-cervical mass 7cm in length. Histological diagnosis may be difficult and may be misdiagnosed as other vascular tumours (Kaposi's sarcoma, hemangiopericytoma).

Aiyer et al (2004) stated that extra-nodal non-Hodgkin's lymphoma of larynx is found in the older age group. It is usually of B-cell type which has a better prognosis than T-cell type. They can present as isolated lesions in larynx or associated with multiple involvement. They are usually found in the supraglottic region of the larynx.

Cohen et al (2004) cited that laryngeal schwannomas were first described by Suchanek in 1925. These were uncommon benign laryngeal tumours presenting as insidious submucosal masses in the supraglottis bringing diagnostic and management challenges to otolaryngologist. These arise from internal branch of superior laryngeal nerve and their differential diagnosis includes chondromas, adenomas, mucoceles, laryngoceles, lipomas and neurofibromas. Hence a biopsy is essential for diagnosis and in planning treatment.

Jaiswal and Hoang (2004) cited a case of combined primary squamous and small cell carcinoma of the larynx, the so-called composite tumour of the larynx. Although major risk factors for developing these composite tumours of the larynx are thought to be similar to other more common neoplasms of the larynx, the treatment and prognosis are different. The supraglottic region is the most frequently involved site.

Madani-Kermani (2004) cited that mucoepidermoid carcinoma is a neoplasm of salivary gland origin and its laryngeal occurrence is extremely rare. This malignant tumour is composed of two distinct cell types, the epidermoid and mucus cells. Prognosis is largely dependent on histologic pattern. To date less than 100 cases have been reported in literature and it occurs between ages 45 to 75 years. Males are more commonly affected. It originates from submucosal glands and may attain a size upto 5 cm in greatest dimension. The supraglottic area is the most common site involved.

Maheshwari et al (2004) stated that primary rhabdomyosarcoma of the larynx is an extremely rare malignancy and the available literature on this medical oddity is in the form of isolated case reports only. They described an 18-year-old boy who presented with a smooth mass in left hemi larynx extending down from the aryepiglottic fold and also involving the glottic region. Mobility of left vocal cord was impaired. Histopathological examination of the endoscopic biopsy material revealed hyperplastic squamous epithelium with intact basement membrane. The tumour was mainly submucosal and sheets of tumour cells invaded submucosal connective tissue. A final diagnosis of embryonal rhabdomysarcoma was made.

Maheshwari et al (2004) cited a case of primary angiosarcoma of larynx which is an extremely rare malignancy. Only 21 cases have so far been reported in the literature. It is reported equally in male and female; more often seen in the middle aged patients. It can affect any site in the larynx. It usually spreads by hematogenous route and pulmonary metastases are the most common site of distant spread.

Munjal et al (2004) described a case of malignant fibrous histocytoma of larynx (MFH). It was first described by Kaufmann and Stout (1961) as a diverse group of benign and malignant tumours that are believed to have a common origin from tissue histocyte. The laryngeal origin is a rare presentation among head and neck MFHs.

Rossini et al (2004) documented a case of renal cell carcinoma (RCC) metastatic to the larynx. Metastatic lesions of larynx are uncommon and often simulate primary cancers. Men are more frequently affected with a male:female ratio less than 2:1. RCC represents approximately 3% of all adult cancers and 23% of patients have distant metastases at the time of diagnosis. RCC metastates to the head and neck have a prevalence of 15.2%. The supraglottic region appears to the most common laryngeal subsite for RCC metastatic lesions compared with glottic and subglottic involvement.

According to Varshney et al (2004) verrucous carcinoma was first delineated as a clinicopathologic entity by Ackerman in 1948 which is an uncommon variant (1 or 2%) of laryngeal squamous cell carcinoma. The typical lesion is a pale, warty, fungating, locally aggressive, ulcerated tumour attached by a broad base, is well circumscribed and it is clearly demarcated from adjacent mucosa. Metastasis is rare, but growth is inexorable in the untreated patient. The tumour can result in the patients' death. Microscopically verrucous carcinoma tends to be broadly based with an irregular surface sometimes thrown into papillary fronds. The surface is usually heavily keratinised. The presence of keratin on an irregular moist mucous surface gives the lesion its white, warty, clinical appearance.

Gillenwater et al (2005) studied a small series of patients with moderately differentiated neuroendocrine carcinoma (MDNC) of the larynx and stated that laryngeal MDNC is an aggressive malignancy with frequent regional and distant metastases.

Greene et al (2005) cited that atypical carcinoid is most frequent of neuroendocrine lesions of larynx. The 1991 WHO classification of laryngeal tumours divided neuroendocrine neoplasms into carcinoid, atypical carcinoid, small cell carcinoma and paraganglioma. Clinically, atypical carcinoid has an aggressive course.

Dotto et al (2006) cited that solitary fibrous tumours are relatively rare mesenchymal neoplasms that were originally described as pleural or peritoneal based lesions. Solitary fibrous tumour of larynx presents in men at a mean age of 42 years (29-60 years). Patients are usually non-smokers and clinically develop progressive hoarseness, foreign body sensation, cough or even acute upper airway distress.

Fonseca et al (2006) stated that papillary squamous cell carcinoma is an entity characterized by highly atypical squamous cell proliferation. Stromal invasion is rarely seen. The differential diagnosis of an exophytic or papillary lesion should include verrucous carcinoma and squamous papillomatosis. The importance of the differential diagnosis lies in the diverse prognoses of these lesions.

Formigoni et al (2006) described a case of adult extracardiac rhabdomyoma affecting extrinsic laryngeal muscle. It is considered a benign tumour, rare and originates from wrinkled muscle cells. extracardiac rhabdomyomas can have three histological classifications: adult, fetal and genital. Fetal and adult forms differ in relation to age. The fetal one occurs in children usually less than three years of age and the adult one is more common in fifties, with predilection for males (4:1).

Nerurkar et al (2006) stated that recurrent respiratory papilloma is the most common benign neoplasm of the larynx, both in children and in adults. The aetiology is Human Papilloma Virus (HPV6 & 11), which in 20% of the cases lies in normal epithelium, hence, the high rate of recurrence. These viruses are tissue specific; targeting stratified squamous epithelium of oropharynx, larynx and anogenital region; but not targeting epidermis. Two forms of laryngeal papilloma have been described, an adult onset (AORRP) and the more aggressive juvenile onset (JORRP). Almost 60% to 80% of cases are thought to be childhood onset usually before the age of 3 years. Pregnancy is associated with accelerated papilloma growth with reactivation of latent disease.

Wang et al (2006) cited that salivary gland carcinomas of the larynx are rare and account for less than 1% of laryngeal malignancy. They diagnosed 12 patients with salivary gland carcinoma of larynx out of 1564 patients with laryngeal malignancy. One patient was excluded due to distant metastasis. All the other eleven patients were male, aged between 48 to 84 years, with median age of 65. Three patients were at an early stage (Stage I and II), others were at an advanced stage III or IV. On histopathology, four patients had adenoid cystic carcinoma, three had mucoepidermoid carcinoma and three patients had adenocarcinoma.

Chapter 5. AIMS AND OBJECTIVES

1. To study the clinical aspects of growths of larynx.

2. To study the histopathological patterns of tumours of the larynx.

3. To study the age and sex difference of laryngeal tumours.

4. To study the socioeconomic and occupational differences of laryngeal tumours.

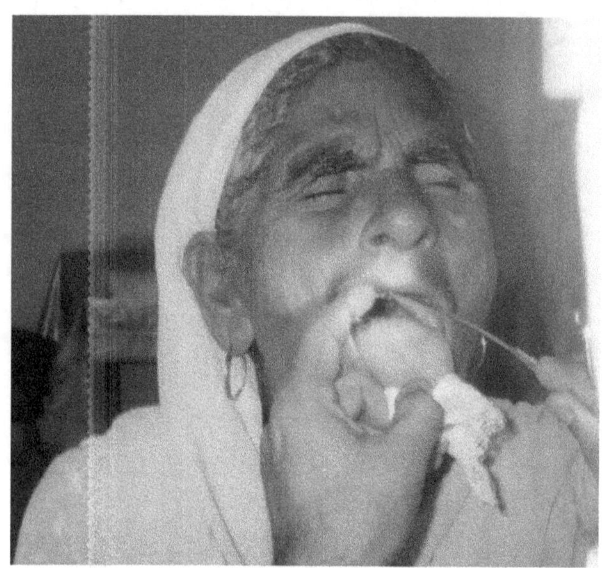

Fig(f) Indirect Laryngoscopy

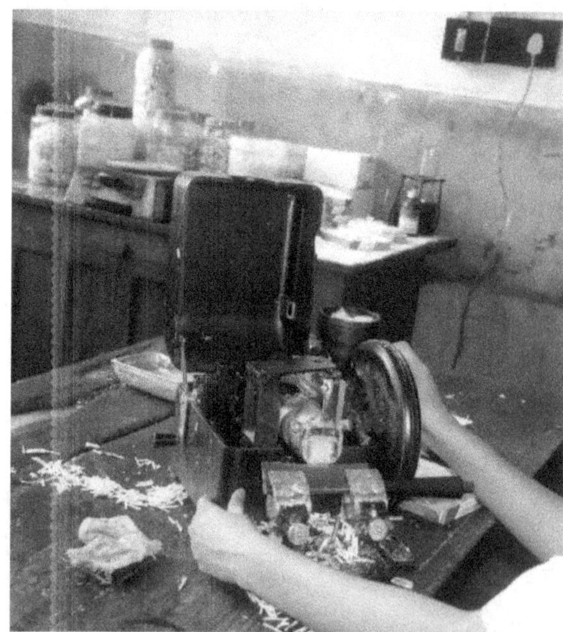

Fig(g) Section Cutting Machine

Chapter 6. MATERIAL AND METHODS

The present study was undertaken on 50 patients clinically diagnosed as cases of tumour of larynx.

The study was conducted in the department of Ear, Nose and Throat (ENT) of the Government Medical College and Rajindra Hospital, Patiala. A complete clinical history of each patient was taken and they were thoroughly examined and investigated according to the proforma enclosed in the appendix.

History

As in all clinical evaluations, the history was the first step in gathering the facts. Following enquiries were made:

- Change in character of voice
- Pain at site
- Difficulty in breathing or swallowing
- Earache
- Coughing up blood or solid material
- Swelling neck
- Weight loss
- Fatigue

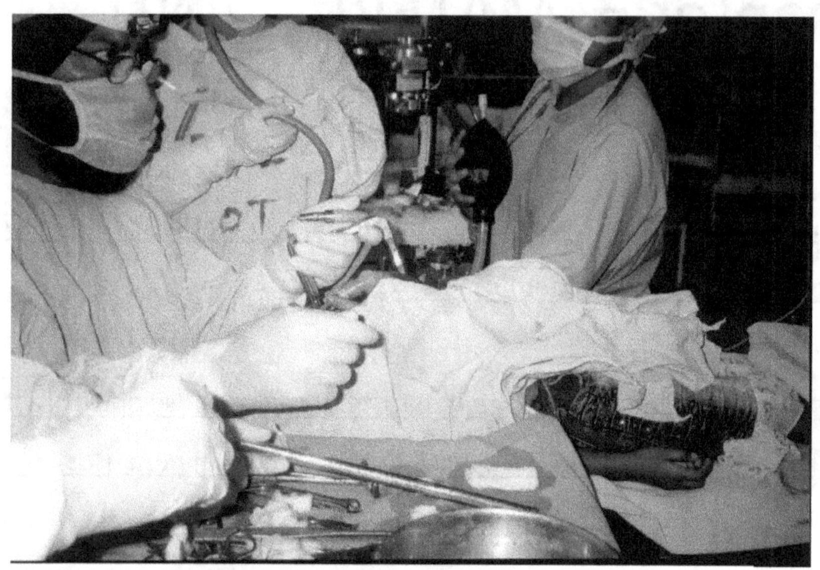

Fig(h) Direct Laryngoscopy under GA

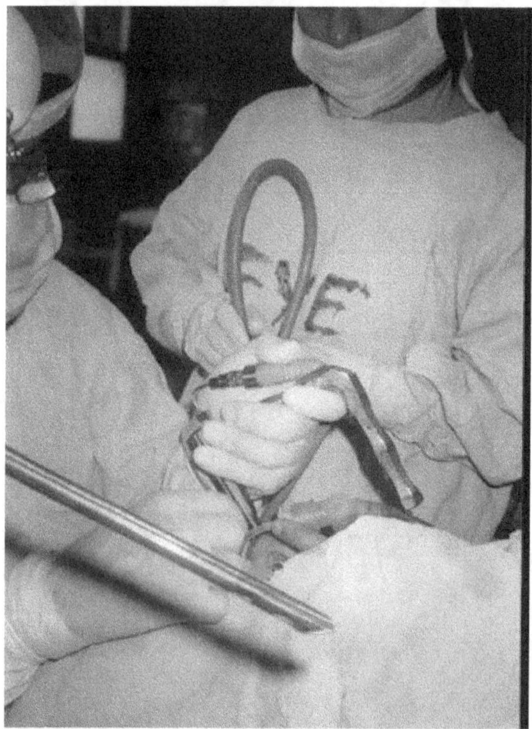

Fig(i) Direct Laryngoscopy

78

Physical examination

When the patient spoke the voice was carefully listened to. This gave an idea of the likely location of the tumour. Thorough head and neck examination was done. This included evaluations of neck mobility, neck masses, direct examination of the oropharynx and epiglottic tip without the aid of instrumentation; and examination of the cranial nerves.

Patients complaining of these symptoms were clinically examined in the Out Door (OPD) department of ENT. Out of these 50 patients suspected of having tumour in the larynx after indirect (mirror) laryngoscopy (Fig f) were admitted in the ward.

These patients were made to undergo direct laryngoscopy (Fig h & Fig i) which was done under local or general anaesthesia. In the cases of apprehensive patients and in children, general anaesthesia was used. The patient was kept fasting overnight. An injection of fortwin and atropine; and viscous oral spray was given 30-45 minutes before laryngoscopy as pre-medication for local anaesthesia. The findings of indirect laryngoscopy were confirmed, the details regarding extent and type of growth were examined; and the biopsy taken from the growth in the larynx was sent to the department of pathology for histopathological examination (Fig g).

Tabulation of cases was done on basis of age, sex, socio-economic status and occupational differences.

Age (years):   0-10, 10-20, 20-30, 30-40, 40-50, 50-60, 60-70

Sex: Male/Female

Socio-Economic Status: Lower class < Rs.1000 pm,

                          Middle class   Rs.1000 to 5000 pm,

                          Upper class > Rs.5000 pm

Occupation: Housewife, Businessman, Farmer, Teacher,

                          Student, Truck driver, Vendor, Worker in

                          hosiery, Labourer

Chapter 7. OBSERVATION AND ANALYSIS

50 patients having tumours of larynx were selected for this study. After thorough ENT examination in the Out Patient Department (OPD) these patients were admitted in the ward for further examination and investigations. The biopsy specimens were examined in the Department of Pathology, Government Medical College and Rajindra Hospital, Patiala for confirming the diagnosis.

The observations are as follows:

50 cases of tumours of larynx were recorded in a period of $2^{1/2}$ years.

Correlation with respect to age, sex, socio-economic status, geographical area and occupational differences was done.

The predisposing factors, symptomatology, histopathological classification and site were also tabulated.

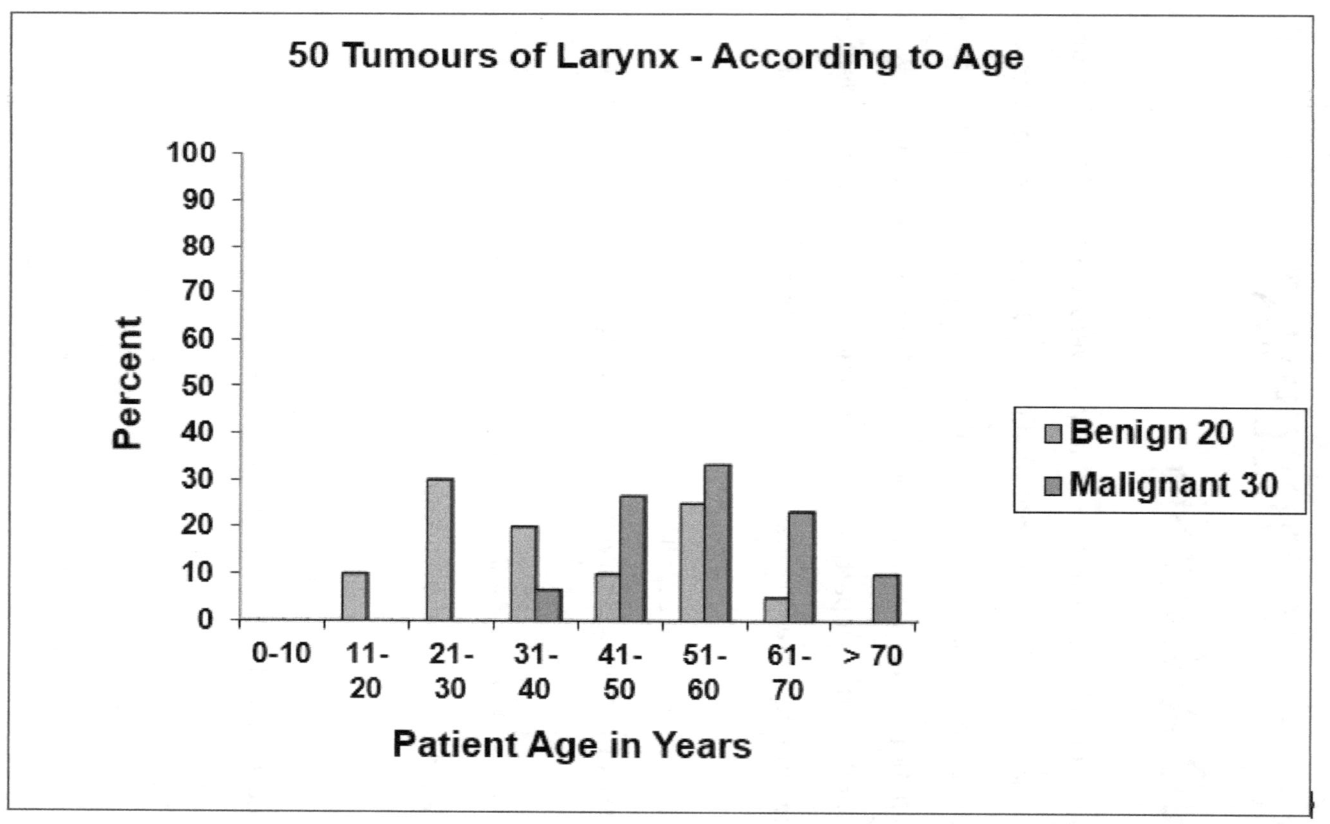

50 Tumours of Larynx - According to Age
Percent
100
90
80
70
60
50
40
30
20
10
0
Benign 20
Malignant 30
0-10
11- 20
21- 30
31- 40
41- 50
51- 60
61- 70
> 70
Patient Age in Years

Age

Table I Benign tumours

Age in Years	No. of Cases	Per. of total (%)
0 – 10	0	0
11 – 20	2	10
21 – 30	6	30
31 – 40	4	20
41 – 50	2	10
51 – 60	5	25
61 – 70	1	5
> 70	0	0
Total cases	**20**	**100**

Age Table II Malignant tumours

Age in Years	No. of Cases	Per. of total (%)
0 – 10	0	0
11 – 20	0	0
21 – 30	0	0
31 – 40	2	6.6
41 – 50	8	26.6
51 – 60	10	33.3
61 – 70	7	23.3
> 70	3	10
Total cases	**30**	**100**

According to the above tables, benign tumours were most common in the third decade (30%) and minimum in the seventh decade (5%). Malignant tumours were reported between the ages of 31 to 80 years with maximum occurrence between the ages of 40 to 70 years. This indicates that young age is less prone to malignant growths.

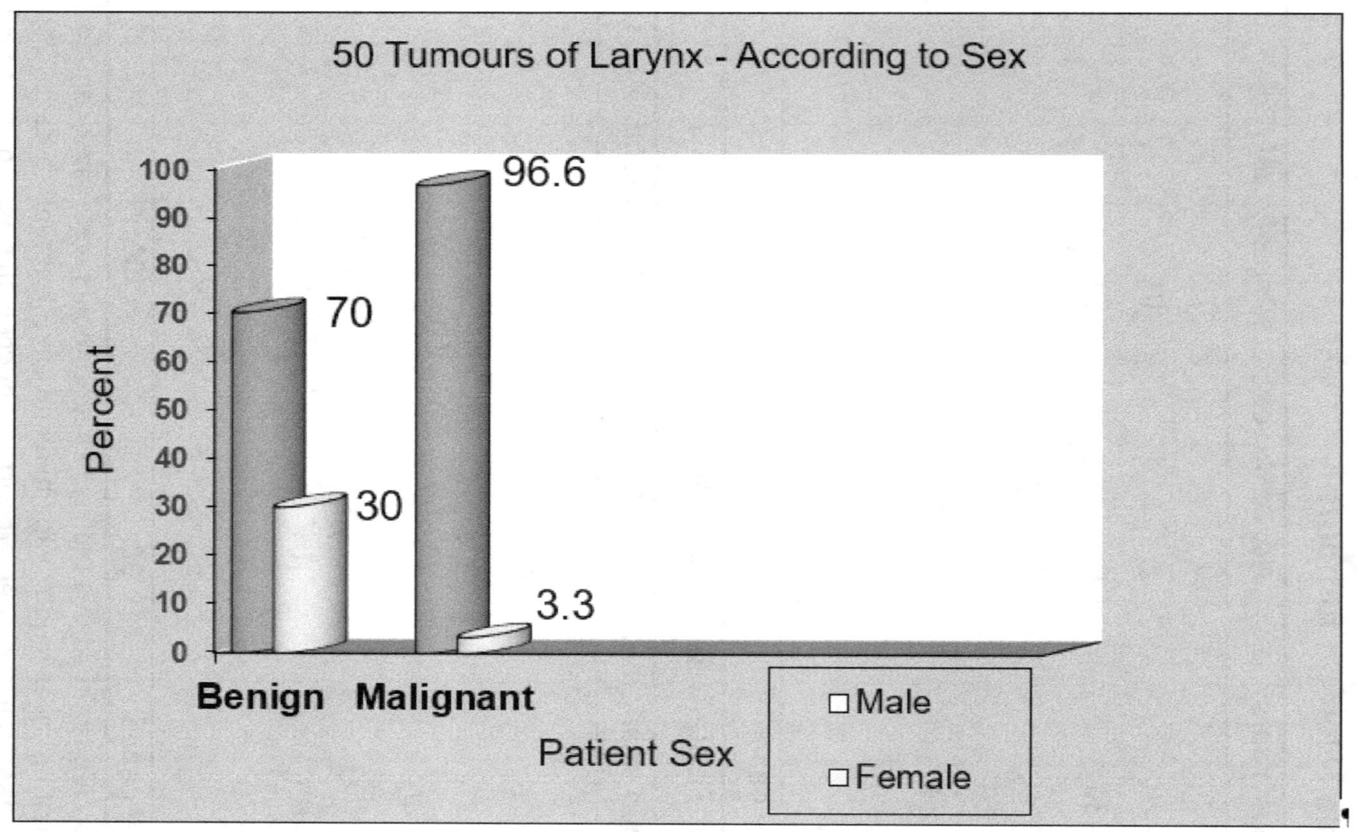

50 Tumours of Larynx - According to Sex
Percent
100
90
80
70
60
50
40
30
20
10
0
70
30
96.6
3.3
Benign
Malignant
Patient Sex
Male
Female

Sex

Table III Benign tumours

Sex	No. of Cases	Per. of total (%)
Male	14	70
Female	6	30
Total cases	**20**	**100**

Sex Table IV Malignant tumours

Sex	No. of Cases	Per. of total (%)
Male	29	96.6
Female	1	3.3
Total cases	**30**	**100**

According to the above tables, both benign as well as malignant tumours were more common in males as compared to females.

Vocal strain, occupation and habits related to smoking and drinking alcohol in the males may have played a role.

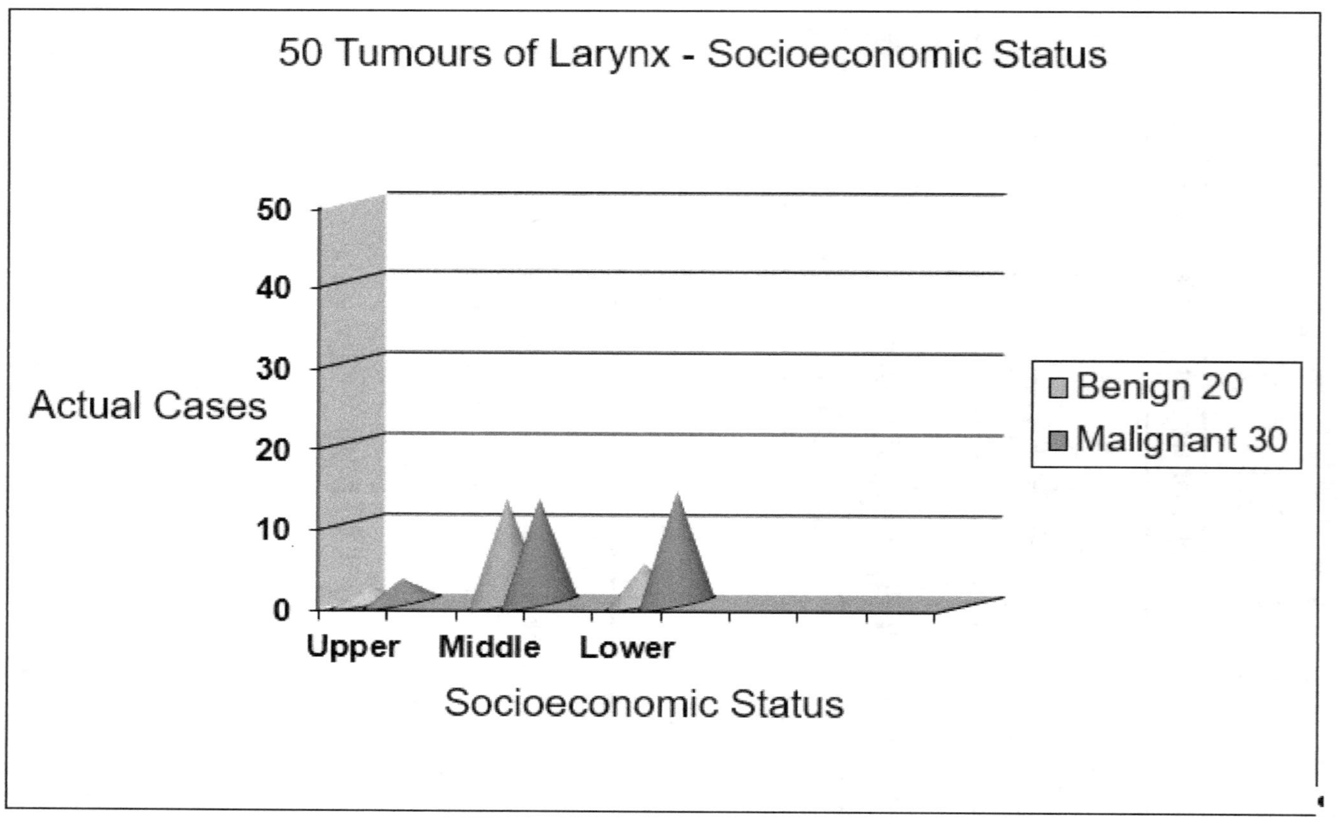

50 Tumours of Larynx - Socioeconomic Status
Actual Cases
50
40
30
20
10
0
Upper
Middle
Lower
Socioeconomic Status
Benign 20
Malignant 30

Socioeconomic status
Table V Benign tumours

Socioeconomic status	*No. of Cases*	*Per. of total (%)*
Upper class	2	10
Middle class	13	65
Lower class	5	25
Total cases	**20**	**100**

Table VI Malignant tumours

Socioeconomic status	*No. of Cases*	*Per. of total (%)*
Upper class	3	10
Middle class	13	43.3
Lower class	14	46.6
Total cases	**30**	**100**

According to above tables the prevalence of benign tumours was more in the middle class (65%) whereas that of malignant tumours was reported more in the lower (46.6%) and middle class (43.3%). Unhygienic conditions, especially carelessness with orodental hygiene and poor nutrition leading to anaemia, play a role in the occurrence of malignant tumours.

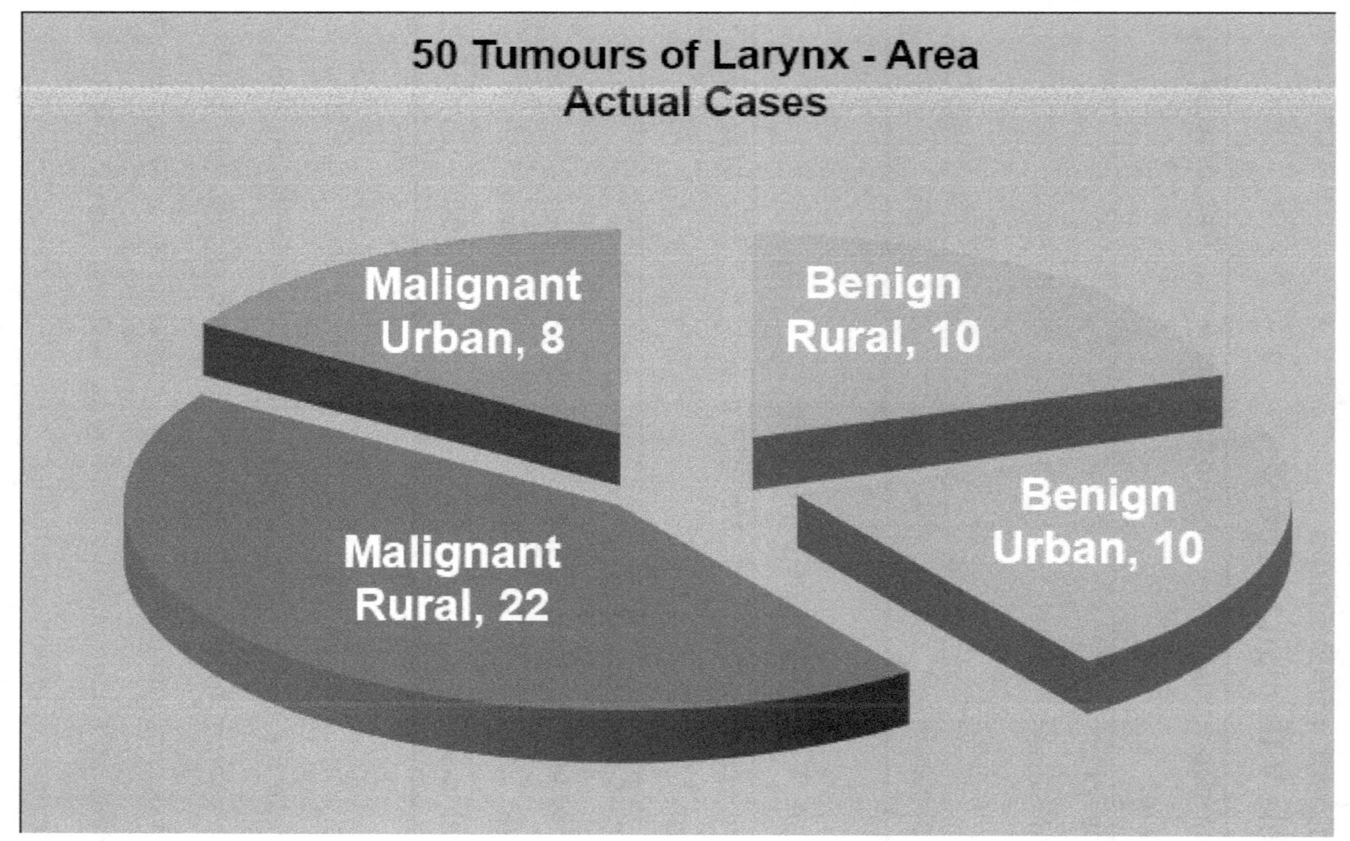

50 Tumours of Larynx - Area
Actual Cases
Malignant
Urban, 8
Benign
Rural, 10
Benign
Urban, 10
Malignant
Rural, 22

Area

Table VII Benign tumours

Area	*No. of Cases*	*Per. of total (%)*
Rural	10	50
Urban	10	50
Total cases	**20**	**100**

Area Table VIII Malignant tumours

Area	*No. of Cases*	*Per. of total (%)*
Rural	22	73.3
Urban	8	26.6
Total cases	**30**	**100**

According to above tables benign tumours were seen equally in rural and urban areas, while malignant tumours were more common (73%) in rural areas.

Addictions such as smoking beedis, chewing tobacco and betel-nut being more common in rural males and use of pesticides in farms can be the cause of higher occurrence of malignant tumours in rural areas.

Notes:
Labourer includes chowkidars
Businessman includes vendors
Skilled includes cobbler, sapera, worker, driver, sevadar, student
White collar includes nurse, retd. teacher, retd. army officer

50 Tumours of Larynx - Occupation

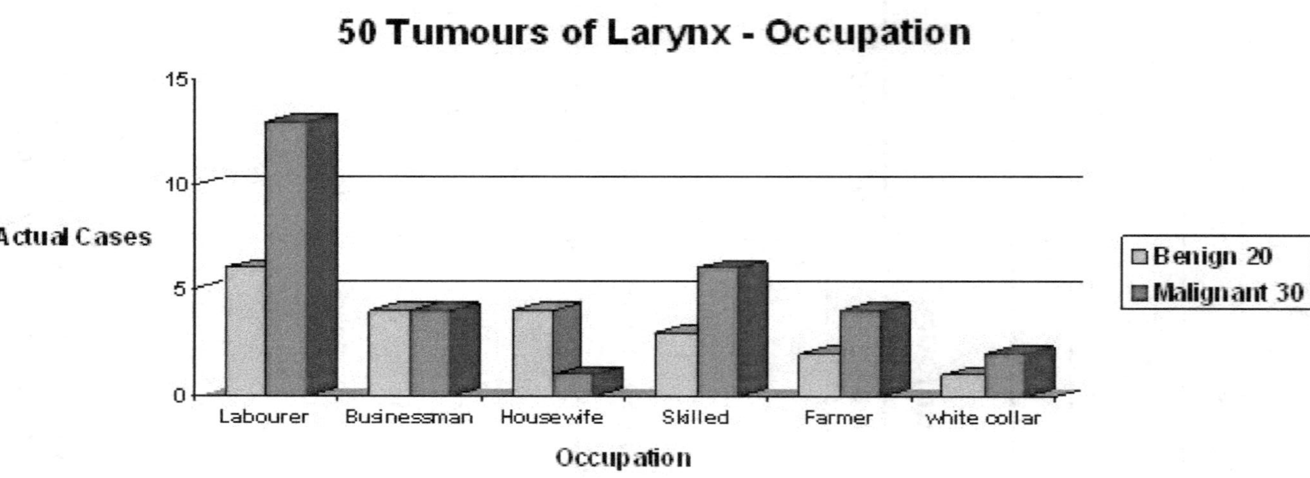

Occupation
Table IX Benign tumours

Occupation	No. of Cases	Per. of total (%)
Housewife	4	20
Businessman	4	20
Teacher	0	0
Student	2	10
Farmer	2	10
Staff Nurse	1	5
Cobbler	1	5
Retired Army Officer	0	0
Labourer	5	25
Chowkidar	1	5
Total cases	**20**	**100**

Occupation Table X Malignant tumours

Occupation	No. of Cases	Per. of total (%)
Housewife	1	3.3
Businessman	3	10.0
Teacher	1	3.3
Sevadar	1	3.3
Farmer	4	13.3
Sapera(Snake charmer)	1	3.3
Skilled Worker	2	6.6
Retired Army Officer	1	3.3
Labourer	11	36.6
Chowkidar	2	6.6
Vendor	1	3.3
Truck Driver	2	6.6
Total cases	**30**	**100**

According to above tables, prevalence of benign tumours was more amongst labourers (25%), followed by business community (20%) and housewives (20%). The business community consisted of shopkeepers or milkmen. Malignant tumours were highest (36.6%) amongst labourers, followed by farmers (13.3%) and businessmen (10%).

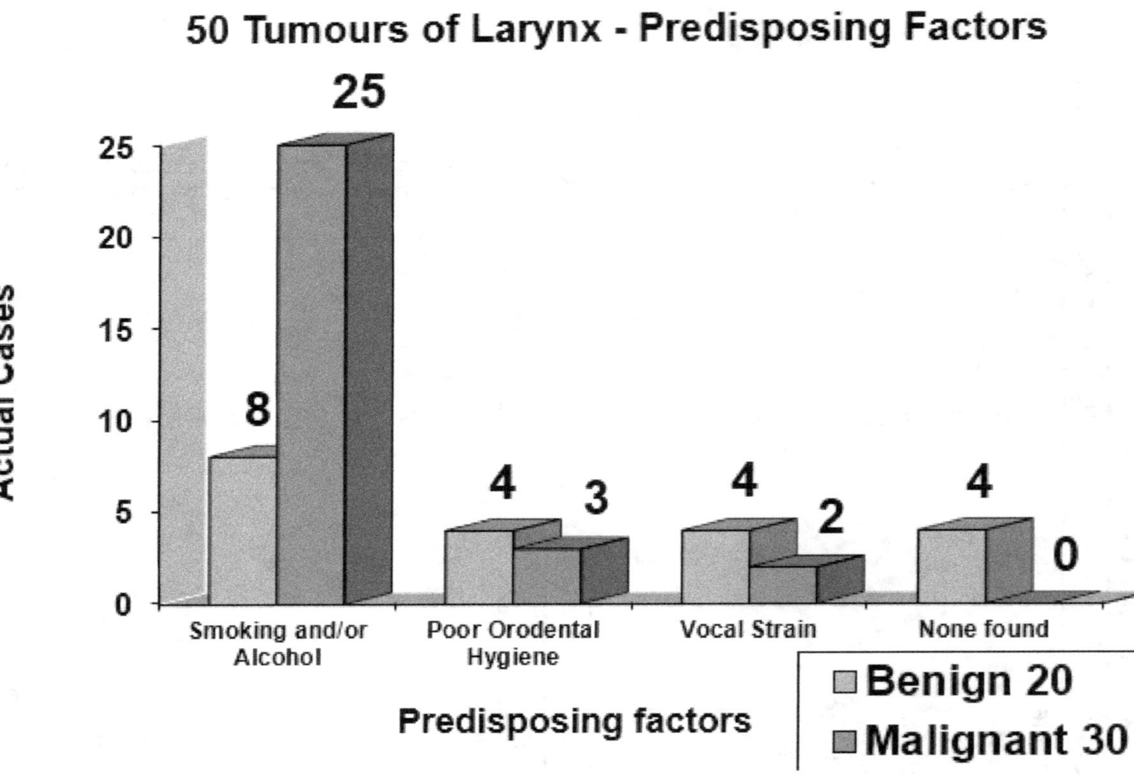

50 Tumours of Larynx - Predisposing Factors
25
Actual Cases
25
20
15
10
8
5
4
4
4
3
2
0
0
Smoking and/or Alcohol
Poor Orodental Hygiene
Vocal Strain
None found
Predisposing factors
Benign 20
Malignant 30

Predisposing Factors
Table XI Benign tumours

Predisposing Factors	No. of Cases	Per. of total (%)
Vocal Strain	4	20
Smoking / tobacco use	5	25
Alcohol use	3	15
Poor orodental hygiene	4	20
No factor found	4	20
Total cases	**20**	**100**

Table XII Malignant tumours

Predisposing Factors	No. of Cases	Per. of total (%)
Vocal Strain	2	6.6
Smoking / tobacco & alcohol use	22	73.2
Alcohol use	3	10
Poor orodental hygiene	3	10
Plummer Vinson Syndrome	0	0
Asbestos dust exposure	0	0
Total cases	**30**	**100**

According to above tables smoking played the main role in benign growths (25%). Vocal strain (20%) and poor orodental hygiene (20%) were other significant predisposing factors. In 20% cases no predisposing factor could be ascertained.

The main predisposing factor (73.2%) for malignant growths was smoking, tobacco chewing and alcohol abuse.

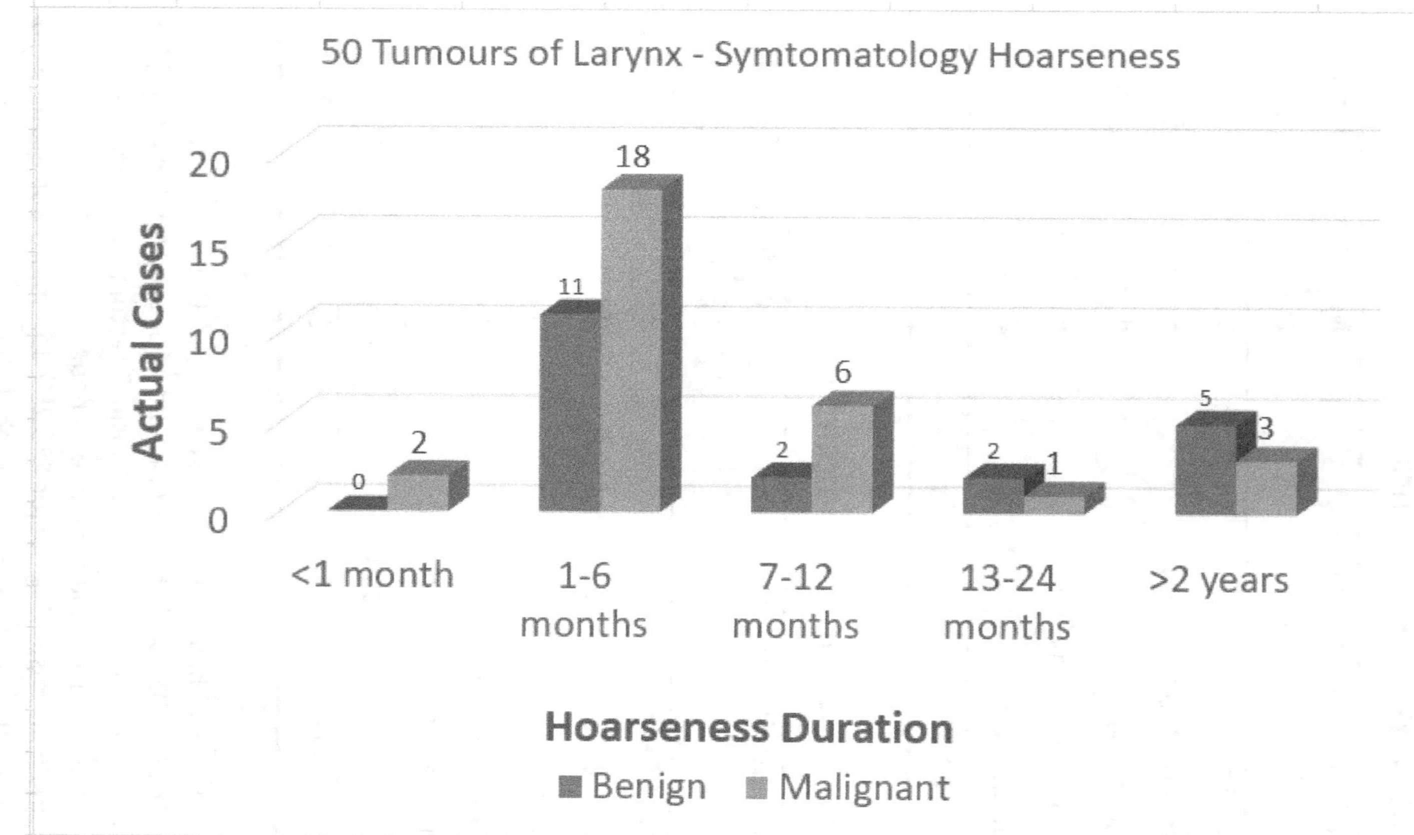

50 Tumours of Larynx - Symtomatology Hoarseness
Actual Cases
20
15
10
5
0
0
2
11
18
2
6
2
1
5
3
<1 month
1-6 months
7-12 months
13-24 months
>2 years
Hoarseness Duration
Benign
Malignant

Symptomatology
Table XIII Benign tumours

Symptomatology	*Period*	*No. of Cases*	*Per. of total %*
Hoarseness	Less than 1 month	0	-
	1 – 6 months	11	-
	7 – 12 months	2	-
	13 – 24 months	2	-
	More than 2 years	5	-
	Hoarseness cases	**20**	**100**
Difficulty in breathing (dyspnoea)	Less than 1 month	1	-
	1 – 6 months	3	-
	7 – 12 months	1	-
	13 – 24 months	0	-
	More than 2 years	0	-
	dyspnoea cases	**5**	**25**
Difficulty in swallowing (dysphagia)	Less than 1 month	0	-
	1 – 6 months	1	-
	7 – 12 months	1	-
	13 – 24 months	0	-
	More than 2 years	0	-
	dysphagia cases	**2**	**10**

Other associated symptoms	Cough	5	25
	Sore Throat	5	25
	Loss of Appetite	0	0
	Foreign body sensation in throat	3	15

Note: Due to multiple symptoms of one patient the data herein will exceed 100%

Table XIV Malignant tumours

Symptomatology	Period	No. of Cases	Per. of total %
Hoarseness	Less than 1 month	2	-
	1 – 6 months	18	-
	7 – 12 months	6	-
	13 – 24 months	1	-
	More than 2 years	3	-
	Hoarseness cases	**30**	**100**
Difficulty in breathing (dyspnoea)	Less than 1 month	2	-
	1 – 6 months	7	-
	7 – 12 months	2	-
	13 – 24 months	0	-
	More than 2 years	1	-
	dyspnoea cases	**12**	**40**

Difficulty in swallowing (dysphagia)	Less than 1 month	2	-
	1 – 6 months	11	-
	7 – 12 months	1	-
	13 – 24 months	1	-
	More than 2 years	0	-
	dysphagia cases	**15**	**50**
Other associated symptoms	Cough and Sore throat	6	20
	Sticking of food in throat	6	20
	Pain in ear	1	10
	Mass in neck	5	16.6
	Fever	1	3.3
	Haemoptysis	5	16.6
	Weight loss	8	26.6
	Appetite loss	6	20

Note: Due to multiple symptoms of one patient the data herein will exceed 100%.

According to above tables, **hoarseness** was the main symptom with which all patients of benign and malignant tumours presented. Most of them had complained of hoarseness for more than six months. Five patients of benign tumours and twelve patients of malignant tumours presented with difficulty in breathing (dyspnoea). Nine cases of malignant tumours had emergency tracheostomy done due to respiratory distress and one case of benign tumour had to undergo tracheostomy due to severe respiratory distress (Fig j).

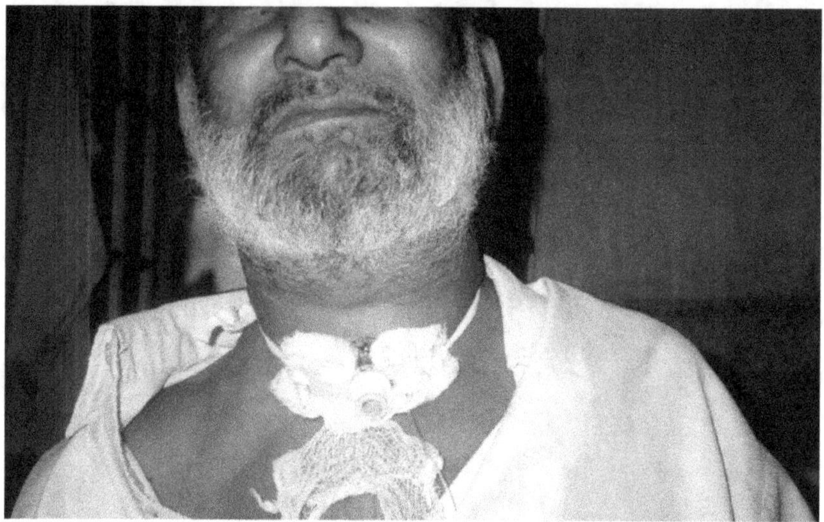

Fig(j) Tracheostomy tube in situ

Difficulty in swallowing (dysphagia) was seen in two patients of benign tumours and fifteen patients of malignant tumours. While most of the patients of benign tumours had one or two symptoms, patients with malignant tumours had multiple symptoms.

Five patients of malignant tumours had associated lymph node enlargement in neck. Five cases of malignant tumours complained of blood in sputum (haemoptysis).

So the patients with tumours of larynx present late due to slow progression of symptoms.

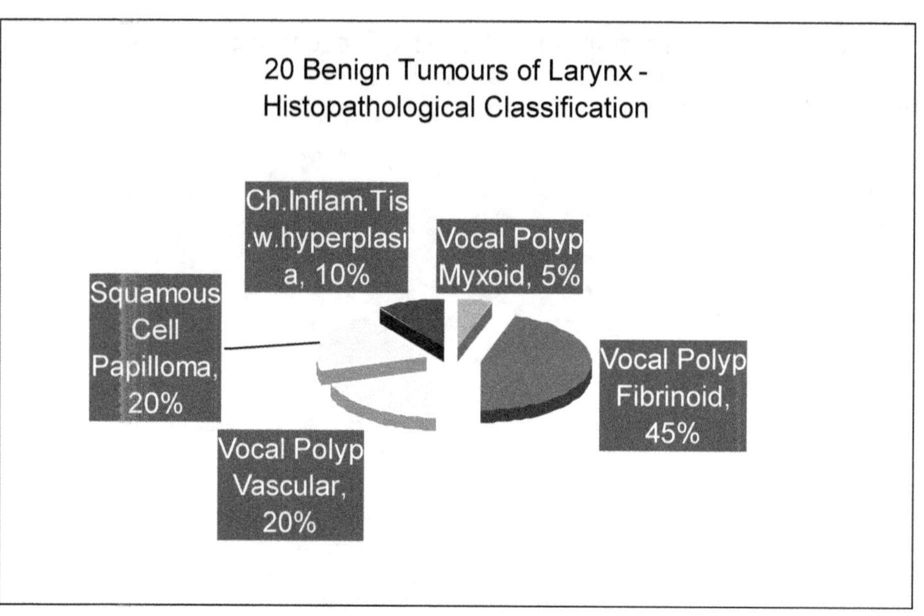

20 Benign Tumours of Larynx - Histopathological Classification
Ch.Inflam.Tis.w.hyperplasia, 10%
Vocal Polyp Myxoid, 5%
Squamous Cell Papilloma, 20%
Vocal Polyp Fibrinoid, 45%
Vocal Polyp Vascular, 20%

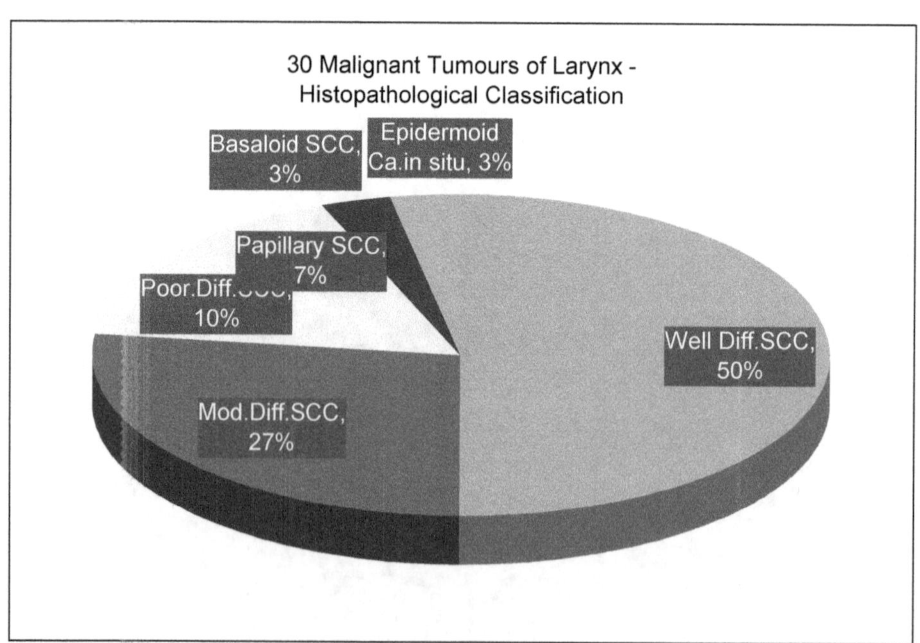

30 Malignant Tumours of Larynx - Histopathological Classification
Basaloid SCC, 3%
Epidermoid Ca.in situ, 3%
Papillary SCC, 7%
Poor.Diff.SCC, 10%
Well Diff.SCC, 50%
Mod.Diff.SCC, 27%

Histopathological Classification
Table XV Benign tumours

Histopathological diagnosis	No. of Cases	Per. of total (%)
Vocal Polyp – Myxoid	1	5
Vocal Polyp - Fibrinoid	9	45
Vocal Polyp - Vascular	4	20
Squamous cell papilloma	4	20
Chronic Inflammatory tissue with hyperplasia and mild dysplasia	2	10
Total cases	**20**	**100**

Table XVI Malignant tumours

Histopathological diagnosis	No. of Cases	Per. of total (%)
Well differentiated Squamous Cell Carcinoma (SCC)	15	50
Moderately differentiated SCC	8	26.6
Poorly differentiated SCC	3	10
Papillary SCC	2	6.6
Basaloid SCC	1	3.3
Epidermoid Ca in situ	1	3.3
Total cases	**30**	**100**

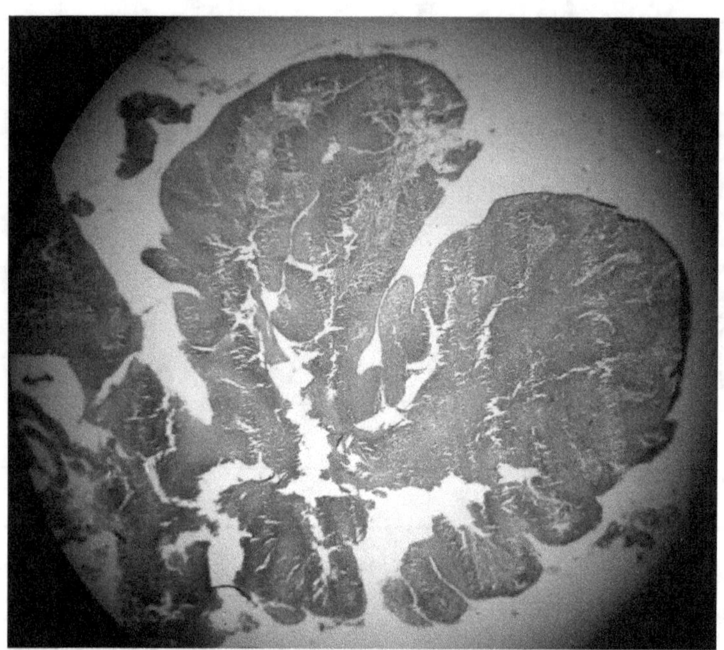

Fig(k) Tracheostomy Squamous Cell Papilloma Larynx (H&E 10X)

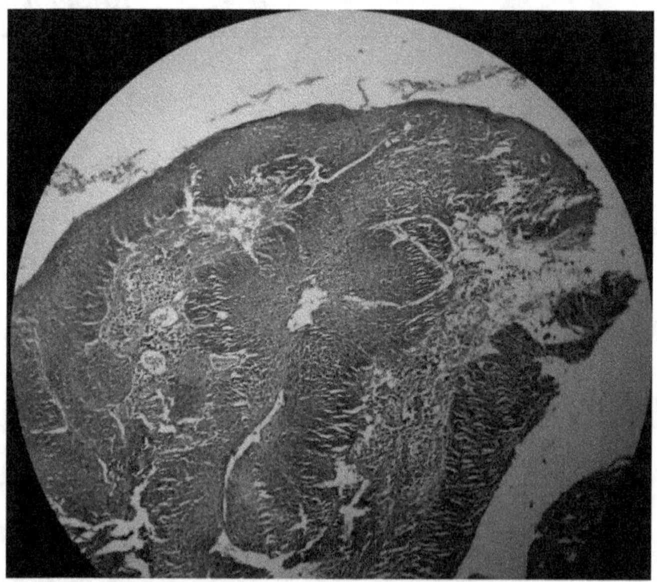

Fig(l) Tracheostomy Squamous Cell Papilloma Larynx (H&E 40X)

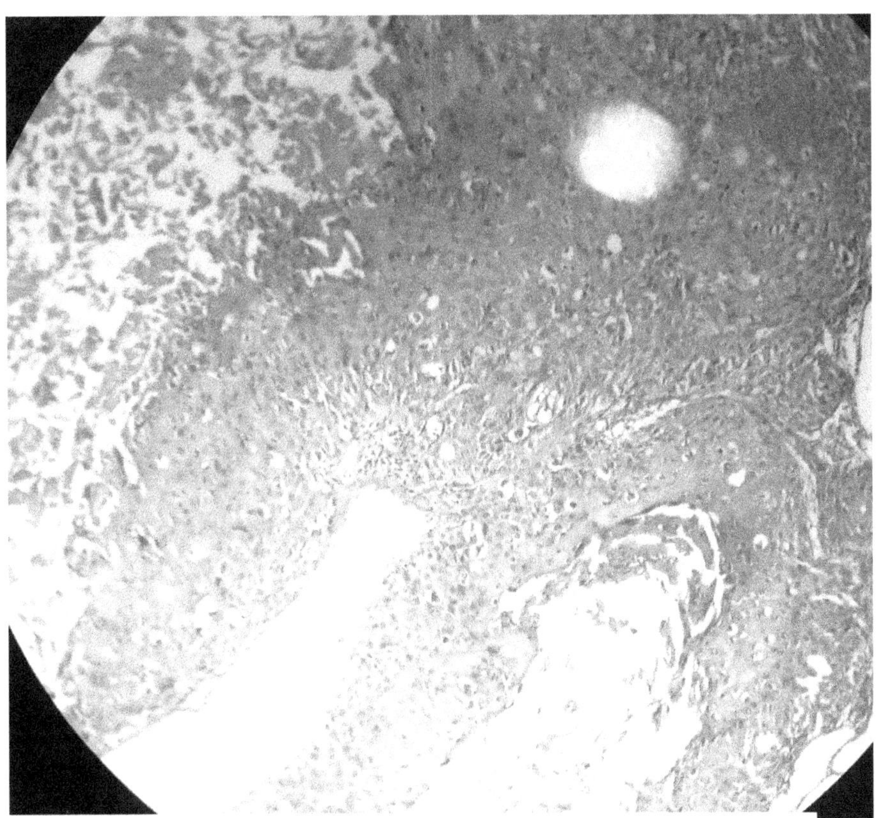

Fig(m) Well Differentiated SCC (H&E 40X)

According to Histopathological tables xv and xvi, the ratio of benign to malignant tumours in the larynx is 2:3. The most common benign tumour of larynx was the vocal polyp. Out of 14 cases of vocal polyp, histopathologically, one case was of myxoid variety, nine were of fibrinoid type and four were vascular.

Squamous cell papilloma of larynx (Fig k & Fig l) was seen in two cases. Chronic inflammatory infiltrate with hyperplasia and mild dysplasia was seen in two cases.

Out of the 30 cases of squamous cell carcinoma, fifteen were well differentiated (Fig m), eight were moderately differentiated and three were poorly differentiated. There were two cases of papillary squamous cell carcinoma, one case of basaloid squamous cell carcinoma and one case of epidermoid carcinoma in situ.

50 Tumours of Larynx – Site Classification

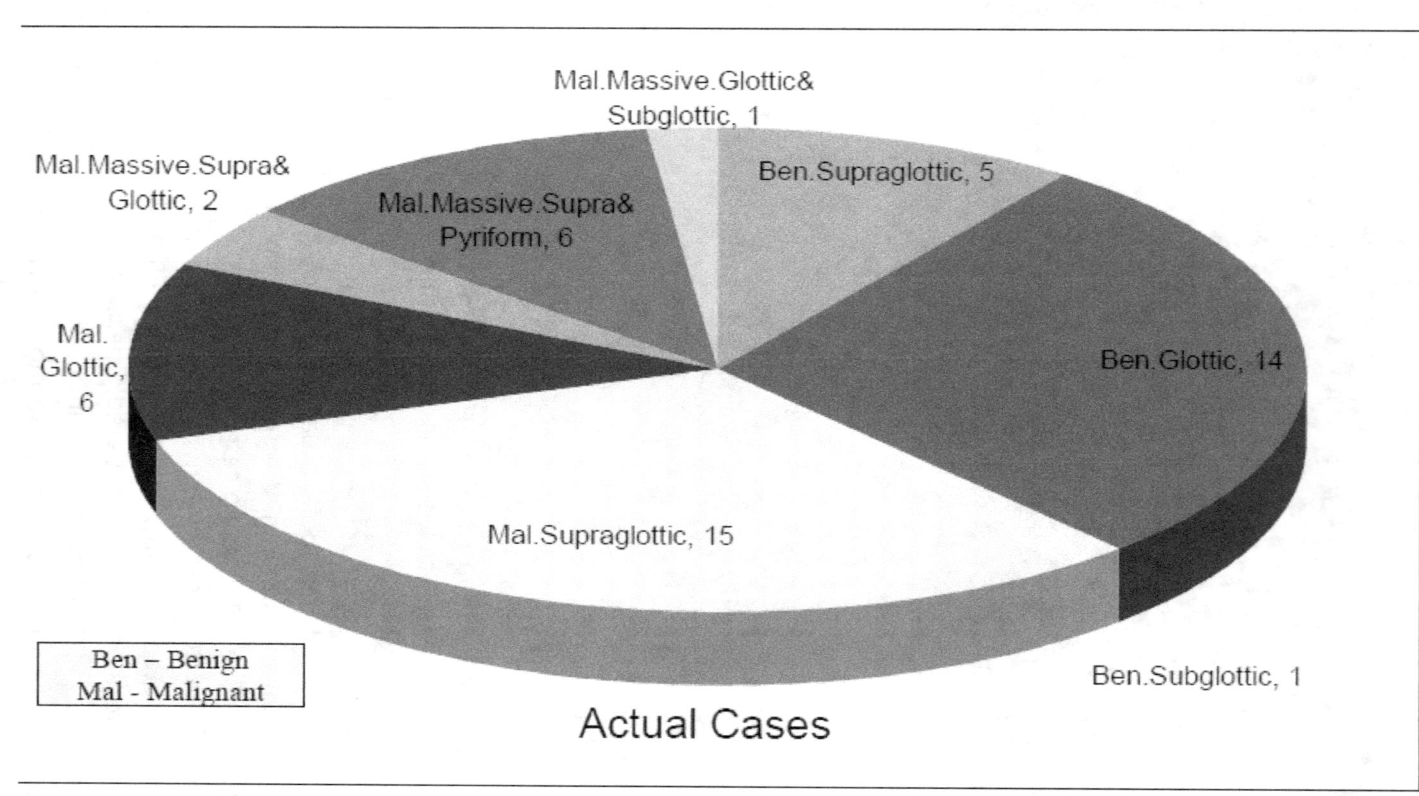

50 Tumours of Larynx – Site Classification

Site of Laryngeal Tumour

Table XVII Benign tumours

Site of growth	No. of Cases	Per. of total %
Supraglottic	5	25
Glottic	14	70
Subglottic	1	5
Total cases	**20**	**100**

Table XVIII Malignant tumours

Site of growth	No. of Cases	Per. of total %
Supraglottic	15	50
Glottic	6	20
Subglottic	0	0
Massive growth involving supraglottic and glottic regions	2	6.6
Massive growth involving supraglottic region and pyriform fossae	6	20
Massive growth involving glottic and subglottic regions	1	3.3
Total cases	**30**	**100**

According to the above tables, the majority of the benign tumours in the larynx arose from the glottic region (70%) followed by that of supraglottis (25%). Only in one case benign growth was detected in the subglottic region.

Patients with malignant tumours had most of them limited to supraglottic region (50%). Some patients had extensive growths involving more than one region, e.g. supraglottic and pyriform fossae (20%), supraglottic and glottic (6.6%), glottic and subglottic (3.3%).

Chapter 8. DISCUSSION

Tumours of the larynx are usually detected early due to dysphonia, i.e. change in voice, but the early and precise diagnosis of cancer of the larynx is still a challenge. Many times it is difficult to determine whether a patient has or does not have cancer of the larynx, but as the disease progresses, the diagnosis can be made more easily and confidently.

All available methods of study should be utilized to make the diagnosis as early as possible. When it has been established that a cancer is present in these regions, it must be determined what structures it involves and its precise extent. In this way, a more effective treatment regime can be selected for the patients.

50 patients with tumours of larynx were studied at the ENT Department of Government Medical College and Rajindra Hospital, Patiala.

Various factors discussed were:

1. Age and Sex distribution
2. The relationship with Rural and Urban origin of the patients
3. The Occupation of the patients and their Socioeconomic Status
4. The Signs and Symptoms
5. Aetiological factors
6. Localization of tumours in diverse sites of the larynx

Biopsy was taken in all the patients and histopathological examination was done in the Department of Pathology, Government Medical College, Patiala.

Observations of the present study are being discussed herein with observations recorded by other workers in this field.

AGE

Benign tumours were most common in the third decade (30%) and minimum in the seventh decade (5%) in this study.

Holinger et al (1968) in a study of 174 patients with laryngeal papilloma found the incidence was slightly more in the age group above 13 years as compared to below 13 years of age. Dinsdale et al (1990) stated that benign laryngeal neoplasms especially lipomas occur more commonly in the seventh decade of life.

So the findings of benign tumours are consistent with Holinger et al (1968), but not with Dinsdale et al (1990).

Table XIX Comparative studies of Age of benign tumours

Author (year)	Age (years)
Holinger et al (1968)	>13
Dinsdale et al (1990)	60 to 70
Present study (2007)	20 to 30

Table XX Comparative studies of Age of malignant tumours

Author (year)	Age (years)
Rowley and Boles (1972)	51 to 70
Shirley (1997)	33 to 91
Cocks et al (1999)	41 to 60
Thompson et al (1999)	27 to 89
Present study (2007)	40 to 70

In the present study the cases of malignant tumours were reported between the ages of 31 to 80 years with maximum occurrence between the ages of 40 to 70 years. Rowley and Boles (1972) in a study of 118 supraglottic laryngeal carcinomas found that 74% were in their 6th to 7th decades of life. Shirley (1997) stated that malignant laryngeal tumours tend to increase with age, average age of diagnosis being 66 years and have been diagnosed over an age range of 33 to 91 years. Cocks et al (1999) stated that cancer of the larynx can occur at any age with mean presentation at 50 to 60 years for men and a decade younger for women. Thompson et al (1999) in a study of 104 patients including 79 men and 25 women of exophytic and papillary squamous cell carcinoma of larynx; found the mean age to be 61 years (the range being from 27 to 89 years).

The present findings are more or less consistent with the studies of Shirley (1997), Cocks et al (1999) and Thompson et al (1999).

<u>SEX</u>

According to present study the occurrence of both benign as well as malignant tumours was higher in males as compared to females. The male to female ratio was 7:3 (i.e. 2.3:1) in case of benign tumours and 29:1 in case of malignant tumours.

Holinger et al (1968) mentioned that laryngeal papilloma had equal sex distribution in pre-puberty age and predominance of males in post-puberty. Arnold et al (1987) found that vocal cord polyp afflicted males of 30 to 50 years of age and twice as frequently as females.

The present study for benign tumours is consistent with those of Holinger et al (1968) and Arnold et al (1987).

Table XXI

Comparative studies of Sex ratio of benign tumours

Author (year)	*Male:Female*
Arnold et al (1987)	2:1
Present study (2007)	2.3:1

Table XXII

Comparative studies of Sex ratio of malignant tumours

Author (year)	*Male:Female*
Kaufman and Burke (1997)	5:1
Cocks et al (1999)	8:1

Thompson et al (1999)	3.2:1
Thompson and Gannon (2002)	3.6:1
Bakshi et al (2004)	15:1
Goiato (2005)	32:1
Present study (2007)	29:1

Kaufman and Burke (1997) found that most patients who develop laryngeal squamous cell carcinomas are males with the male to female ratio being 5:1. Cocks et al (1999) stated that cancer of the larynx predominantly affects males with a male to female sex ratio of 8:1. Thompson et al (1999) in a study of 104 cases of exophytic and papillary squamous cell carcinomas found that 79 of these were in males and 25 of these were in females. Thompson and Gannon (2002) in a study of 111 cases of laryngeal tumours found a male to female ratio of 3.6:1. Bakshi et al (2004) in a study of 690 cases of carcinoma larynx found that 647 patients were males and 43 were females. Goiato (2005) in a study of 66 cases of laryngeal cancer found that 64 of these were males and they represented 97% of the cases, the rest being females.

In case of malignant tumours, male:female ratio is high as compared to Kaufman and Burke (1997), Cocks et al (1999), Thompson et al (1999); and Thompson and Gannon (2002). It is consistent with that of Bakshi et al (2004) and Goiato (2005).

According to the socioeconomic background, the patients were broadly divided into three groups viz. upper, middle and lower. In present study the prevalence of benign tumours was more in the middle class, while malignant tumours were common in both the lower and middle classes.

Maier et al (1992) in a study of 164 male patients with squamous cell carcinoma of larynx found that this cancer was more common in the peoples of low socioeconomic status. Smith (2003) stated that low socioeconomic status is associated with cancers of the larynx. Bakshi et al (2004) in a study of 690 cases of laryngeal carcinoma found that 60% were from the low socioeconomic status, 25% belonged to the middle class and the remaining 15% belonged to the high class. Goiato (2005) in a study of 66 patients of laryngeal cancer found that it was more prevalent in peoples of low socioeconomic status.

In case of benign tumours, no other study could be found to correlate present findings with socioeconomic status. However for malignant tumours this study is consistent with the above studies that malignant tumours are more common in peoples from low socioeconomic status.

According to present study the occurrence of benign tumours was the same for patients belonging to rural as well as urban areas. However the prevalence of malignant tumours was more in peoples from the rural areas.

Smith (2003) stated that tobacco-related cancers like those of the larynx tend to be related to the population living in rural surroundings. Bakshi et al (2004) in their study of 690 patients found that 78% were rural and the remaining 22% were from urban regions. Goiato (2005) also found in a study of 66 cases of cancer of the larynx that it was more prevalent in peoples from rural areas.

The present study is also in line with these studies.

Table XXIII

Comparative studies of Residential Area of malignant tumours

Author (year)	*Rural, Urban*
Bakshi et al (2004)	78%, 22%
Present study (2007)	73.3%, 26.6%

<u>OCCUPATION</u>

The maximum occurrence of benign tumours was found in labourers (25%), followed by businessmen (20%) and housewives (20%) in present study.

No other study could be found to correlate benign tumours with occupation.

Table XXIV

Comparative studies of Occupation of malignant tumours

Author (year)	Occupation
Bakshi et al (2004)	Farmers (45%), Labourers (39%)
Present study (2007)	Farmers (13.3%), Labourers (36.6%)

Maier et al (1992) in a study of 164 patients of cancer of the larynx found that 90% of the cases were blue collar workers, most of them working in dirty or dusty jobs. Bakshi et al (2004) in a study of 690 cases of carcinoma of larynx found that of these 45% were farmers and 39% were labourers. Goiato (2005) in a study pertaining to risk factors of laryngeal cancers carried out in Turkey found higher risk factors among watchmen, drivers and building construction workers. *In present study out of 30 cases of malignant tumours of the larynx, 36.6% were labourers, 13.3% farmers and 10% businessmen. So it is consistent with the above studies that cancer of the larynx is more common in blue collar workers than in white collar jobs.*

In present study, smoking turned out to be the most common (25%) predisposing factor, followed by vocal strain (20%) and poor orodental hygiene (20%) in the case of benign tumours.

Rains and Ritchie (1984) found that papilloma is a lesion occurring at any age but is more common in children and associated with human papilloma virus (HPV 11) in most cases.

The present study could not correlate any case with human papilloma virus for benign tumours.

Table XXV

Comparative studies of main Predisposing factor of malignant tumours

Author (year)	Smoking and/or Alcohol Abuse
Rowley and Boles (1972)	70%
Thompson et al (1999)	83.7% and 47%
Bakshi et al (2004)	87.8% and 75%
Present study (2007)	73.2%

Rowley and Boles (1972) in a review of 118 laryngeal carcinomas done over ten years found that 70% were heavy smokers (10 to 20 cigarettes a day) and 7% were light to moderate smokers (less than 10 cigarettes a day). Maier et al (1992) in a study of 164 cases found that smoking and drinking alcohol increase the dose-dependent risk of laryngeal cancer. Kaufman and Burke (1997); and Adams and

Maisel (1998) also stated that tobacco and alcohol abuse are associated with increased risk of laryngeal cancer. Thompson et al (1999) in a study of 104 cases of laryngeal cancer found that 87 patients were using tobacco and 49 patients smoked and/or drank alcohol. Bakshi et al (2004) in a study of 690 cases of laryngeal cancer found that smoking was a predisposing factor in 87.8% of the cases and additionally or otherwise alcohol consumption was in 75% of the cases. Goiato (2005) in a study of 66 cases of malignancy of larynx found that tobacco smoking and alcohol use are the highest risk factors for laryngeal cancer. In the present study in case of malignant tumours, smoking and tobacco chewing and alcohol use (73.2%) were the most common predisposing factors.

The present study is consistent with above studies in so far as smoking is the predominant predisposing factor in malignancies of larynx and, that of alcohol use being an added factor.

Some other studies are also mentioned here:

Stell and McGill (1973) reported exposure to asbestos dust as a predisposing factor for cancer of the larynx. Maier et al (1992) also found exposure to asbestos as a predisposing factor in 7.5% of their patients in a study of 164 patients.

In the present study no exposure to asbestos could be established.

In present study, hoarseness was the earliest and main presenting symptom in both benign as well as malignant growths. While most patients with benign tumours had only one symptom, patients with malignant tumours had associated symptoms like dyspnoea, dysphagia, cough, haemoptysis and secondaries in the neck.

Thompson et al (1999) in a study of 104 cases of squamous cell carcinoma of larynx found that patients had hoarseness at presentation. Kumar et al (2004) stated that carcinoma of the larynx manifests clinically by persistent hoarseness and later produces pain, dysphagia and haemoptysis. Bakshi et al (2004) in their study of 690 cases of carcinoma of larynx found that hoarseness was the most common complaint. Other complaints were sore throat, neck nodes and haemoptysis.

So present study is consistent with the above studies that hoarseness is the most common complaint for cases of tumours of larynx.

<u>CLASSIFICATION OF TUMOURS CLINICALLY AND</u>

<u>HISTOPATHOLOGICALLY ACCORDING TO THEIR NATURE</u>

<u>BENIGN / MALIGNANT</u>

A vocal polyp is covered with stratified squamous epithelium and may exhibit a variety of changes in the stroma which include oedema fibrosis, increased vascularity, haemorrhages and hyaline changes. Thus on the basis of differing histological changes, vocal polyps were divided into fibrinoid, vascular and myxoid polyps.

Another type of benign growth detected was squamous cell papilloma which is a benign epithelial neoplasm formed by stratified squamous epithelium. These tumours are usually exophytic. The papilloma is a true neoplasm that grows as a soft succulent, raspberry like friable excrescence; usually on true vocal cords.

Squamous cell carcinoma was the most common malignant tumour detected in the larynx. Out of the 26 cases of squamous cell carcinoma, fifteen were well differentiated, eight were moderately differentiated and three were poorly differentiated. A squamous cell carcinoma is an invasive tumour that shows evidence of squamous differentiation.

In present series there were two cases of papillary squamous cell carcinoma, one case of basaloid squamous cell carcinoma and one case of epidermoid carcinoma in situ. Papillary squamous cell carcinoma shows finger-like projections with fibrovascular cores or broad based bulbous growth with rounded projections and limited fibrovascular cores; overlying squamous epithelium is malignant; usually no/limited surface keratinisation. Basaloid squamous cell carcinoma shows typical areas of squamous cell carcinoma (invasive and in situ) with nests or cords of small crowded cells with minimal cytoplasm, hyperchromatic nuclei, comedonecrosis, prominent hyalinization and peripheral palisading, small cystic spaces and mitotic activity.

Table XXVI
Comparative studies of Histopathology of laryngeal tumours

Author (year)	Benign:Malignant
Arnold et al (1987)	1:10
Present study (2007)	2:3

In the present study the ratio of benign to malignant tumours was 2:3. Out of the benign tumours, 70% were vocal polyps, 20% were squamous cell papilloma and 10% were chronic inflammation.

Arnold et al (1987) found that papilloma was the most frequent benign tumour of the larynx with the ratio of benign to malignant tumours being 1:10. Cocks et al (1999) found that the majority of benign laryngeal lesions are vocal cord polyps. Nerurkar et al (2006) reported that recurrent respiratory papilloma (RRP) is the most common benign neoplasm of larynx both in children and in adults.

The ratio of benign to malignant tumours in present study was 2:3 as compared to that of Arnold et al (1987) of 1:10. It was consistent with Cocks et al (1999) who showed that vocal cord polyp was the most common benign tumour. It differed from the study of Nerurkar et al (2006) who reported that RRP is the most common benign neoplasm of larynx.

Table XXVII Comparative studies of frequency of SCC amongst laryngeal malignancy

Author (year)	Incidence (Percentage)
Kaufman and Burke (1997)	>90%
Kumar et al (2004)	95%
Jaiswal and Hoang (2004)	99%
Bakshi et al (2004)	96%
Domanowski (2006)	96%
Wang et al (2006)	99%
Present study (2007)	100%

The present findings showed that in cases of malignant tumours 100% were squamous cell carcinoma (SCC). Out of these 50% were well differentiated SCC, 26.6% were moderately differentiated SCC, 10% were poorly differentiated SCC, 6.6% were papillary SCC and 3.3% were basaloid SCC. There was only one case of epidermoid in situ.

Kaufman and Burke (1997) stated that SCC of the larynx accounts for over 90% of laryngeal cancers. Kumar et al (2004) stated that 95% of all laryngeal carcinomas are typical SCC. Jaiswal and Hoang (2004) stated that out of all primary laryngeal carcinomas, 99% are SCC. Bakshi et al (2004) in a study of 690 cases of laryngeal malignancy found that 69% were non-keratinizing SCC and 27% were keratinizing SCC. Greene et al (2005) cited that in the larynx, SCC is the most common malignant tumour. Domanowski (2006) cited that 96% of laryngeal carcinomas are SCC. Wang et al (2006) stated that SCC accounts for 99% of all primary laryngeal carcinomas.

The present study is also in line with the above studies.

CLINICAL CLASSIFICATION ACCORDING TO <u>**SITE**</u>

The site and extent of tumour in all cases was determined by indirect and direct laryngoscopy, X-Ray soft tissue neck and chest X-Ray postero-anterior (PA) views. In present study, the majority (70%) of the benign tumours were glottic, 25% were supraglottic and only 5% were subglottic.

Arnold et al (1987) cited that vocal polyps predominantly occur over anterior half of the vocal cords and may be bilateral in 20% of the cases.

The present study is consistent with the study of Arnold (1987) that the most common site of benign vocal polyps is the glottic area.

Table XXVIII

Comparative studies of Site of malignant tumours

Author (year)	Supraglottic, Glottic, Subglottic, Transglottic %
Thompson et al (1999)	30, 46, 3, 21
Bakshi et al (2004)	56, 17, 3.6, 13
Present study (2007)	50, 20, 0, 30

In the case of malignant tumours, 50% were supraglottic, 20% glottic, 30% transglottic and none subglottic in present study.

Thompson et al (1999) studied 104 cases of exophytic and papillary SCCs of larynx out of which 30% were supraglottic, 46% glottic, 3% subglottic and 21% transglottic. Bakshi et al (2004) in a study of 690 cases of laryngeal malignancy found that 56% of tumours were supraglottic, 17% glottic, 3.6% subglottic and 13% transglottic tumours.

The malignant tumours of the larynx occur more commonly in the supraglottis which is consistent with the studies of Bakshi et al (2004) but not with that of Thompson et al (1999). The present study is in line with both the above studies that subglottis is the least common site.

Chapter 9. SUMMARY AND CONCLUSION

Fifty cases of tumours of larynx detected on indirect laryngoscopy were selected from Ear, Nose and Throat (ENT) Outpatients Department of Government Medical College and Rajindra Hospital, Patiala. These were recorded in a period of $2^{1/2}$ years.

Every patient was admitted to the ENT ward and subjected to a detailed clinical history and general physical examination. Routine investigations like Haemoglobin (Hb), Bleeding Time (BT), Clotting Time (CT) and special investigations like X-Ray soft tissue neck and chest X-Ray were done. Direct laryngoscopy was conducted on all patients. Wherever possible the growth was excised or a biopsy taken which was subjected to histopathological examination.

The conclusions drawn from the present study are as follows:

From history it was noted that benign tumours were most common in the third decade (30%) and minimum in the seventh decade (5%). Malignant tumours were most prevalent in the age group 40 to 70 years.

The incidence of both benign (7:3) and malignant (29:1) tumours was higher in males than in females.

Most of the patients with benign tumours of larynx belonged to the middle class (65%) as far as socioeconomic status was concerned. The majority of the patients of malignant tumours of larynx belonged to the lower (46.6%) or middle classes (43.3%).

Regarding occupation, the highest prevalence of benign (25%) and malignant (36.6%) tumours was amongst labourers. In benign tumours, other occupations involved were businessmen (20%) and housewives (20%). In cases of malignant tumours, other occupations were farmers (13.3%) and businessmen (10%).

Various predisposing factors were noted. In benign tumours the main predisposing factor was smoking and tobacco use (25%). Other predisposing factors were poor orodental hygiene (20%) and vocal strain (20%). In cases of malignant tumours, smoking with alcohol abuse was the main predisposing factor (73.2%) while poor orodental hygiene (10%) and vocal strain (6.6%) were found in fewer cases.

Hoarseness was the main presenting symptom. Only one case of benign tumour presented with dyspnoea and had to get tracheostomy done. In case of malignant tumours there were other associated symptoms like dyspnoea, dysphagia, sore throat and cough. In nine cases of malignant tumours, emergency tracheostomy had to be done. Eight cases had weight loss, six cases had appetite loss and five cases each had haemoptysis and mass neck as associated complaints.

The most common benign tumour was the vocal polyp (70%). All cases of malignant tumours were squamous cell carcinoma (100%) out of which 50% were well differentiated, 26.6% were moderately differentiated and 10% were poorly differentiated. There were two cases of papillary SCC and one of basaloid SCC. There was only one case of epidermoid carcinoma in situ (3.3%).

Patients with benign tumours had involvement of one site in the larynx, especially the vocal cords (70%). Most cases (50%) of malignant tumours were supraglottic, 30% showed transglottic involvement and 20% were glottic.

BIBLIOGRAPHY

Adams GL, Maisel RH. Malignant tumours of the larynx and hypopharynx In: Otolaryngology, Head and Neck Surgery, Cummings CW, Fredrickson JM, Harker LA, Krause CJ, Schuller DE, editors. 3rd ed. St. Louis; Mosby. 1998. 2130.

Ahluwalia H, Gupta SC, Singh M, Mishra V, Singh PA, Walia DK. Spectrum of Head-Neck Cancers at Allahabad. Indian J Otolaryngol and Head neck Surg 2001; 53(1):16-21.

Ahrens W. Commentary: Socioeconomic status: more than a confounder? Int J Epidemiol 2004; 33:1-2.

Aiyer RG, Soni G, Chougule S, Unnikrishnan, Nagpal T. Extranodal Non-Hodgkin's Lymphoma of Larynx. Indian Journal of Otolaryngology and Head and Neck Surgery 2004; 56(4):298.

Arnold WJ, Laissue JA, Friedmann I, Naumann HH. Larynx In: Diseases of the Head and Neck, Georg Thieme Verlag, Stuttgart 1987; 8:8-13.

Bakshi J, Panda NK, Sharma S, Gupta AK, Mann SBS. Survival Patterns in treated cases of carcinoma larynx in North India – A 10 years follow up study. Indian J of Otolaryngology and Head and Neck Surg 2004; 56(2):99-103.

Barnes L, Ferlito A, Wenig BM. Laryngeal Paragangliomas. A review and report of a single case. J Laryngol Otol 1997; 111:197-8.

Berge JK, Kapadia SB, Myers EN. Osteosarcoma of the Larynx. Arch Otolaryngol Head Neck Surg 1998; 124(1):207-10.

Cocks H, Quraishi M, Morgan D, Bradley P. Leiomyosarcoma of the larynx. Otolaryngol Head Neck Surg 1999; 121:643-6.

Cohen S, Sinacori JT, Courey MS. Laryngeal schwannoma: Diagnosis and Management. Otolaryngol Head Neck Surg 2004; 130:363-5.

Dinsdale RC, Manning SC, Brooks DJ, Vuitch F. Myxoid laryngeal lipoma in a juvenile. Otolaryngol Head Neck Surg 1990; 103(4):653-7.

Domanowski G. Malignant Tumours of the Larynx In: Head and Neck Oncology, eMedicine from webMD, Coleman JA, Talavera F, Calhoun KH, Slack, Meyers AD, editors. eMedicine World Medical Library 2006; Section 1 to 10.

Dotto JE, Ahrens W, Lesnik DJ, Kowalski D, Sasaki C, Flynn S. Solitary Fibrous Tumour of the larynx: A case report and review of the literature. Archives of Pathology and Laboratory Medicine 2006; 130(2):213-6.

Esposito ED, Motta S, Cassiano B, Motta G. Occult lymph node metastases in supraglottic cancers of the larynx. J Otolaryngology - Head and Neck Surgery 2001; 253-7.

Fonseca AS, Chone CT, Crespo AN, Altemani A. Laryngeal papillary carcinoma with unexpected evolution: case report. Sao Paulo Medical Journal 2006; 124(3):158-60.

Formigoni GG, Fortes FSG, Wiikmann C, Sennes LU, Carneiro PC. Adult Extracardiac Rhabdomyoma compromising the Extrinsic Laryngeal Muscles. International Archives of Otorhinolaryngology 2006; 10(1).

Fung EK, Neuhauser TS, Thompson LD. Hodgkin-like transformation of a marginal zone B-cell lymphoma of the larynx. Ann Diagn Pathol 2002; 6:61-6.

Gillenwater A, Lewin J, Roberts D, El-Naggar A. Moderately Differentiated Neuroendocrine Carcinoma (Atypical Carcinoid) of the Larynx: A Clinically Aggressive Tumour. Laryngoscope 2005; 115(7):1191-5.

Goiato MC, Fernandes AUR. Risk factors of laryngeal cancer in patients attended in the oral oncology centre of Aracatuba. Braz J Oral Sci 2005; 4(13):741-4.

Greene L, Brundage W, Cooper K. Large cell neuroendocrine carcinoma of the larynx: a case report and a review of the classification of this neoplasm. Journal of Clinical Pathology 2005; 58:658-61.

Holinger PH, Schild JA, Maurizi DG. Laryngeal papilloma: review of etiology and therapy. Laryngoscope 1968; 78(9):1462-74.

Hucumenoglu S, Celik N, Erdem G, Kocaturk S. Papillary Adenocarcinoma of the Epiglottis. Turkish Journal of Medical Sciences 2002; 32(2):185-7.

Jaiswal VR, Hoang MP. Primary Combined Squamous and Small Cell Carcinoma of the Larynx. Arch Pathol Lab Med 2004; 128:1279-81.

Jeannon J, Stafford FW, Soames JV, Wilson JA. Altered MUC1 and MUC2 glycoprotein expression in laryngeal cancer. Otolaryngol Head Neck Surg 2001; 124:199-202.

Kaufman JA, Burke AJ. The Etiology and Pathogenesis of Laryngeal Carcinoma In: The Otolaryngologic Clinics of North America, Current Concepts in Laryngeal Cancer I, 1997; 30(1):1-13.

Khalil H, Naraghi A, Denton K, Baldwin D. Paraganglioma of the Larynx Presenting as a Neck Mass. The Internet Journal of Otorhinolaryngology 2003; 2(2).

Kumar V, Abas AK, Fausto N. In: Robins and Cotran's pathologic basis of disease. 7th ed. India: Saunders; 2004. 786-7.

Lee L, Fang T, Li H, Lee K. Adenoid cystic carcinoma of the supraglottic mimicking a laryngeal cyst. Otolaryngol Head Neck Surg 2003; 129:157-8

Lin S, Hsu C, Jan Y. Primary laryngeal melanoma. Otolaryngol Head Neck Surg 2001; 125:569-70.

Loos BM, Wienke JA, Thompson LD. Laryngeal Angiosarcoma: A clinicopathologic study of five cases with a review of the literature. Laryngoscope 2001; 111:1197-1202.

Madani-Kermani SZ. Mucoepidermoid carcinoma of the Larynx: Report of a rare laryngeal tumour. Acta Medica Iranica 2004; 42(2):149-50.

Maheshwari GK, Baboo HA, Gopal U, Wadhwa MK. Primary Rhabdomyosarcoma of the Larynx. Indian Journal of Otolaryngology and Head and Neck Surgery 2004; 56(2):138.

Maheshwari GK, Baboo HA, Patel MH, Gopal U, Wadhwa K. Primary Angiosarcoma of the Larynx. Turkish Journal of Cancer 2004; 34(4):166-8.

Maier H, Gewelke U, Dietz A, Heller W. Risk factors of cancer of the larynx: Results of the Heidelberg case – control study. Otolaryngol Head Neck Surg 1992; 107(4): 577-82.

Maurizi M, Cadoni G, Ottaviani F, Rabitti C, Almadori G. Verrucous Squamous cell carcinoma of the larynx: diagnostic and therapeutic considerations. European Archives of Oto-Rhino-Laryngology 1996; 253(3):130-5.

Munjal M, Sood N, Shah BS, Malhotra V. Malignant Fibrohistocytoma of the Larynx. Indian Journal of Otolaryngology and Head and Neck Surgery 2004; 56(4):289.

Nerurkar N, Kalel K, Pathania V, Bradoo R. Recurrent Respiratory Papilloma in Pregnancy. Bombay Hospital Journal 2006; 48(1):187-90.

Orlandi A, Fratoni S, Hermann I, Spagnoli LG. Symptomatic laryngeal nodular chondrometaplasia: a clinicopathological study. Journal of Clinical Pathology 2003; 56:976-7.

Parker JA. Sarcomas of the larynx In: Grand Rounds Archive BCM Bobby R Alford Department of Otolaryngology – Head and Neck Surgery; 1993.

Pernick N. Larynx and hypopharynx In: Pathology Outlines.com; Crookston K, Cubilla AL, DePond WD, Perunovic B, Rakozy CK. Reviewers. Bingham Farms, Michigan 2006.

Pham TV, Lannigan FJ. Paediatric laryngeal carcinoma: case report, literature review and possible role of agent orange. Australian Journal of Oto-Laryngology 2001; 4(2):136-9.

Rains AJH, Ritchie HD. The Larynx In: Bailey and Love's Short Practise of Surgery. 19th ed. Great Britain: Hazell Watson and Viney Ltd; 1984. 591-93.

Robin PE, Olofsson J. Tumours of the Larynx In: Laryngology and Head and Neck Surgery. Hibbert J, 6th ed. Great Britain:Heinemann International; 1997. 1-9.

Rossini M, Bolzoni A, Piazza C, Peretti G. Renal Cell Carcinoma metastatic to the larynx. Otolaryngol Head Neck Surg 2004; 131:1029-30.

Rowley NJ, Boles R. Supraglottic carcinoma: a 10-year review at the University Hospital. Laryngoscope1972; 82(7):1264-72.

Sasaki CT. Anatomy and development and physiology of the larynx In: PART 1 Oral cavity, pharynx and esophagus, Goyal R, Shaker R, editors. Nature Publishing Group; GI Motility Online 2006; doi:10.1038/gimo7.

Sasaki CT, Isaacson G. Functional Anatomy of the Larynx In: Aspiration and Swallowing Disorders. The Otolaryngologic Clinics of North America 1988; 21(4): 595-612.

Sharma K, Duggal KK, Bal MS. Neurilemmoma of Larynx. IJO & HNS 1995; 47(3):210.

Shaw H. Tumours of the Larynx In: Scott-Brown's Diseases of the Ear, Nose and Throat, Ballantyne J, Groves J, editors. 4th ed. London; Butterworths. 1979. 421.

Shirley D. Cartilaginous lesions of the Larynx. Grand Rounds Archives BCM Bobby R Alford Department of Otolaryngology – Head and Neck Surgery; 1997.

Simon P. Cancer of the larynx (voice box). Jeevodaya Hospice 2005; V(4):3-4

Smith M. Overview of Cancer in Asia. The Asian Journal of Cancer Care, Oncology Forum, Scientific Communications ltd 2003; 6(1).

Sood S, Carney AS, Quraishi MS, Bradley PJ. Carcinoid Carcinoma of the Larynx. Aust J Oto-Laryngol 1999.

Sorrentino R, Vitiello R, Castelli ML. Angiosarcoma of the larynx. Case report and review of the literature. Acta Otorhinolaryngologica Italica 2003; 23(3):191-3.

Standring S. Neck and Upper Aerodigestive Tract - Larynx In: Gray's Anatomy, Standring S, Berkovitz B, editors. 39th ed. Edinburgh; Elsevier Churchill Livingstone. 2005; 36:633-44.

Stell PM, McGill T. Asbestos and laryngeal carcinoma. Lancet 1973; 2(7826):416-7.

Thomas RL. Non-epithelial tumours of the larynx. Journal Laryngol Otol 1979; 93:1131-41.

Thompson LD, Gannon FH. Chondrosarcoma of the Larynx: A Clinicopathological Study of 111 cases with a review of literature. Am J Surg Pathol 2002; 26:836-51.

Thompson LD, Wenig BM, Heffner DK, Gnepp DR. Exophytic and papillary squamous cell carcinomas of the Larynx: A Clinicopathologic series of 104 cases. Otolaryngology Head and Neck Surgery 1999; 120:718-24.

Thompson LD, Wieneke JA, Miettinen M, Heffner DK. Spindle Cell sarcomatoid carcinomas of the Larynx: A Clinicopathologic study of 187 cases. Am J Surg Pathol 2002; 26:153-70.

Varshney S, Saxena RK, Kaushal A, Singh J, Pathak VP. Verrucous Carcinoma of Larynx. Indian Journal of Otolaryngology and Head and Neck Surgery 2004; 56(1):54-6.

Wang M, Liu C, Li W, Chang S, Chu P. Salivary Gland Carcinoma of the Larynx. J Chin Med Assoc 2006; 69(7):322-5.

Welkoborsky HJ, Sorger K, Moll R, Collo D. Primary Larynx Carcinoid. Case Report and review of the literature. Laryngol Rhinol Otol 1988; 67(11):559-63.

Wenig BM, Heffner K. Liposarcomas of the Larynx and Hypopharynx: A Clinicopathologic study of eight new cases and a review of the literature. Laryngoscope 1995; 105:747-56.

Wenig BM. Lipomas of the Larynx and Hypopharynx: A review of the literature with the addition of three new cases. J Laryngol Otol 1995; 109:353-7.

Wenig BM. Necrotizing sialometaplasia of the Larynx. A report of two cases and a review of the literature. Am J Clin Pathol 1995; 103:609-13.

Wieneke JA, Gannon FH, Heffner DK, Thompson LD. Giant Cell tumour of the Larynx: A Clinicopathologic series of eight cases and a review of the literature. Mod Pathol 2001; 14:1209-15.

Wilkinson III AH, Beckford NS, Babin RW, Parham DM. Extraskeletal myxoid chondrosarcoma of the epiglottis: case report and review of the literature. Otolaryngol Head Neck Surg 1991; 104(1):257-60.

PROFORMA

PROFORMA		
Patients Name	Case No	OPD No
Age	Sex	
Father/Husband Name		CR No
Address	Date of Admission	Date of Discharge
Occupation		
Socioeconomic Status		
Chief Complaints		
	Hoarseness of voice	
	Difficulty in breathing/swallowing	
History of (H/o) Present Illness		
Hoarseness of voice		
	Mode of Onset	
	Constant/Intermittent	
	Onset related with rise/no-rise of temp	
	Diurnal variation	
	Feeling of discomfort – pricking sensation on speaking	
Difficulty in breathing		
	Related with exertion	
	Persisting all the time	
Feeling of foreign body sensation in throat		
Difficulty in swallowing		

	Firstly with solids/semisolids/liquids
	Site of obstruction
	Pain during swallowing
Other Symptoms	
	H/o pain in throat
	H/o irritative or paroxysmal cough with increased expectoration or dry cough
	H/o excessive salivation
	H/o blood in sputum
	H/o foetor breath
	H/o ear pain
	H/o appearance of mass in neck
	H/o loss of appetite
	H/o weight loss
	H/o fever
	H/o palpitation
Past History	
	H/o similar episode in the past
	H/o tuberculosis, hypertension, diabetes
Personal History	
	H/o smoking, hookah, pipe, tobacco, or pan chewing
	H/o alcohol intake – how much and how often
	H/o any drug addiction
Environment	
	Exposure to irritants like dust, fumes, smoke,

	asbestos, etc.		
Family History			
	Similar diseases in family		
	H/o hypertension, tuberculosis, diabetes		
General Physical Examination			
	General Appearance	Fever	
	Anaemia	Cyanosis	
	Jaundice		
Neck			
	Thyroid	Jugular Venous Pressure	
	Lymph nodes		
	If any then		
	Single/Multiple	Matted/Discrete	
	Mobile/Fixed	Size	
	Site		
	Any other mass in the neck		
Examination			
	Pulse	Blood Pressure	Oedema Feet
	Chest Examination	Cardio vascular system	Neurological Examination
Local Examination			
	Ear	Nose	
	Throat	Orodental Hygiene	

		Floor of Mouth
		Palate
		Teeth
		Cheeks
	Pharynx	Nasopharynx
		Oropharynx
	Larynx	External Examination
		Any abnormality in shape
		Laryngeal Crepitus
		Tenderness
Indirect Laryngoscopy		
	Posterior surface of tongue	Valleculae
	Epiglottis	Aryepiglottic folds
	Arytenoids	Post Cricoid area
	Anterior commissure	Pyriform fossae
	False Vocal Cords	True Vocal Cords
	Inter-arytenoid region	Sub-glottic area
If mass in larynx present		
	Size	Site	Shape
	Hyperaemia or Infiltration surrounding the growth	
Direct Laryngoscopy		
	Confirmation of above findings and detailed examination	
Investigations		
Haemoglobin	Bleeding	Clotting Time

	Time	
Total Leucocyte Count		Differential Leucocyte Count
Urine Examination		Erythrocyte Sedimentation Rate
X-Ray soft tissue neck		
X-Ray Chest P-A view		
Biopsy Report		

Now we give the Master Charts. For ease of presentation, these charts are split into headings:
- Age/Sex
- Predisposing Factors
- Other Symptoms
- Lab Investigations

In each chart, the same SN refers to one single patient of the 50 studied.

MASTER CHART Age/Sex

SN	CR. No./ Year	Age in yrs	Sex M/F	Rural/Urban	Occupation	Socioeconomic Status (Class)
1	11883/ 2005	54	M	Rural	skilled worker	Middle
2	20448/ 2005	35	F	Urban	housewife	Middle
3	20314/ 2005	55	M	Rural	labourer	Lower
4	20309/ 2005	20	M	Urban Slum	labourer	Lower
5	21740/ 2005	48	M	Rural	farmer	Middle
6	22158/ 2005	58	M	Urban	Security Guard in SBP	Middle
7	22420/ 2005	55	F	Rural	Housewife	Lower
8	23215/ 2005	25	M	Rural	Milkman	Middle
9	24116/ 2005	32	M	Urban	Chowkidar	Middle
10	24285/ 2005	52	M	Rural	Labourer	Lower
11	24639/ 2005	50	M	Urban	Labourer	Lower

12	24951/ 2005	42	M	Rural	Farmer	Middle
13	25708/ 2005	21	M	Urban	Student	Middle
14	25903/ 2005	42	M	Urban	shopkeep er	Middle
15	27009/ 2005	55	M	Rural	Labourer	Middle
16	27679/ 2005	70	M	Rural	Labourer	Lower
17	28192/ 2005	40	F	Rural	Housewife	Middle
18	28070/ 2005	55	M	Urban	Business man	Upper
19	28518/ 2005	30	F	Urban	Housewife	Middle
20	28381/ 2005	53	F	Rural	Housewife	Middle
21	28857/ 2005	50	M	Urban	Vendor	Lower
22	29256/ 2005	60	M	Rural	Labourer	Lower
23	29467/ 2005	60	M	Rural	Driver	Lower
24	1007/ 2006	50	M	Rural	Shopkeep er	Middle
25	1967/ 2006	42	M	Rural	Farmer	Middle
26	2469/ 2006	73	M	Urban	Labourer	Lower

27	2082/ 2006	85	M	Rural	sevadar	Middle
28	2741/ 2006	61	M	Rural	chowkidar	Middle
29	4528/ 2006	65	M	Rural	Labourer	Middle
30	5104/ 2006	65	M	Rural	Labourer	Lower
31	5268/ 2006	55	M	Urban	Skilled worker	Middle
32	5276/ 2006	48	M	Rural	Farmer	Middle
33	10170/ 2006	40	M	Rural	Sapera	Lower
34	10286/ 2006	85	M	Rural	Shopkeeper	Middle
35	10441/ 2006	60	M	Urban	cobbler	Middle
36	10591/ 2006	60	M	Urban	retired army officer	Upper
37	6549/ 2006	70	M	Urban	Labourer	Lower
38	13549/ 2006	28	M	Rural	Farmer	Middle
39	13767/ 2006	40	F	Urban	staff nurse	Upper
40	14363/ 2006	60	M	Rural	Labourer	Lower
41	15869/ 2006	26	M	Urban	Shopkeeper	Upper

SN		Age	Sex	Residence	Occupation	Class
42	18070/ 2006	50	M	Urban	milkman	Middle
43	18280/ 2006	13	F	Rural	Student	Middle
44	20847/ 2006	65	M	Rural	retired teacher	Upper
45	20651/ 2006	32	M	Rural	Farmer	Middle
46	22371/ 2006	56	M	Rural	Truck Driver	Middle
47	20075/ 2006	65	M	Rural	Labourer	Lower
48	24830/ 2006	62	M	Rural	Labourer	Lower
49	25478/ 2006	25	M	Rural	Labourer	Lower
50	26302/ 2006	45	M	Rural	Labourer	Lower

MASTER CHART contd. Predisposing factors

SN	Predisposing factors	Symptomatology (Duration)		
		Hoarseness	Dyspnoea	Dysphagia
1	voice strain	8 months	1 year	-
2	not known	3 months	3 months	3 months
3	smoking & alcohol intake	20 days	-	-
4	smoking	2 months	-	-
5	smoking & bhuki intake	2 years	25 days	-

6	smoking	9 months	-	-
7	not known	6 months	2 months	-
8	voice strain	8 months	-	-
9	poor orodental hygiene	2 months	-	-
10	smoking	2 months	-	-
11	smoking	2 months	-	-
12	smoking	3 months	-	-
13	not known	since childhood	-	-
14	smoking	6 months	-	-
15	poor orodental hygiene	25 days	-	25 days
16	smoking	1 year	1 month	-
17	poor orodental hygiene	2 months	-	2 months
18	smoking	6 months	-	-
19	poor orodental hygiene	2 months	-	-
20	poor orodental hygiene	2 years	1 year	1 year
21	smoking	2 months	-	1 month
22	smoking	5 months	-	5 months
23	smoking & alcohol intake	3 months	-	4 months
24	smoking	1 year	-	6 months
25	poor orodental hygiene	21/2 years	1 month	-
26	smoking & alcohol intake	3 months	20 days	20 days
27	voice strain	8 months	1 month	-

28	smoking	3 months	-	2 months
29	smoking	1 year	1 month	-
30	alcohol intake	3 years	6 months	-
31	smoking	4 months	6 months	-
32	alcohol intake	2 months	-	2 months
33	smoking & alcohol intake	2 months	2 months	7 months
34	smoking	2 months	-	2 months
35	smoking	many years	20 days	-
36	smoking	4 months	1 month	1 month
37	smoking	3 years	many years	3 months
38	voice strain	3 years	-	-
39	voice strain	2 years	-	-
40	poor orodental hygiene	3 months	-	-
41	alcohol intake	6 months	-	-
42	alcohol intake	3 months	-	-
43	not known	since childhood	-	-
44	alcohol intake	4 months	-	-
45	alcohol intake	5 years	-	-
46	smoking & alcohol intake	9 months	-	-
47	smoking & alcohol intake	6 months	1 year	2 years
48	smoking & alcohol intake	4 months	-	4 months
49	voice strain	6 months	-	-
50	smoking	2 months	-	-

MASTER CHART contd. Other Symptoms

SN	Other symptoms (duration)	Direct Laryngoscopy findings	Clinical classification according to	
			Nature	Site
1	-	fungating growth Rt aryepiglottic fold	malignant	supraglottic
2	-	bilateral vocal nodules	benign	glottic
3	cough & sore throat x 3m	growth on left false vocal cord and pyriform fossa	malignant	supraglottic
4	-	left vocal cord polyp	benign	glottic
5	appetite & weight loss x 3m	ulceroproliferative growth on Rt vocal cord extending to Lt vocal cord	malignant	glottic
6	-	ulcerative growth on Lt vocal cord	malignant	glottic
7	-	left vocal cord polypoydal mass	benign	glottic
8	cough & sore throat x 8m	right false vocal cord nodule	benign	supraglottic
9	-	bilateral vocal nodules	benign	glottic

10	-	globular mass on Rt false vocal cord	benign	supraglottic
11	mass Rt side neck x 9m	growth in Rt vallecula and epiglottis	malignant	supraglottic
12	appetite & weight loss x 3m	growth Rt epiglottis & aryepiglottic fold	malignant	supraglottic
13	-	Rt vocal nodule	benign	subglottic
14	cough & sore throat x 2m	small nodule Rt false vocal cord	benign	supraglottic
15	foreign body sensation in throat x 25days	growth on epiglottis and Lt vallecula	malignant	supraglottic
16	appetite & weight loss x 6m	growth Rt false vocal cord	malignant	supraglottic
17	-	growth Lt arytenoid	malignant	supraglottic
18	cough & sore throat x 6m	ulcerative growth on Lt arytenoid & pyriform fossa	malignant	supraglottic
19	-	bilateral vocal nodules	benign	glottic
20	foreign body sensation throat x 2yr	ulcerative growth Rt arytenoid	benign	supraglottic

21	mass Rt side neck x 1m, foreign body sensation throat x 2m	growth Rt vallecula & epiglottis	malignant	supraglottic
22	mass Rt side neck x 15days	fungating growth Rt epiglottis & pyriform fossa	malignant	supraglottic
23	weight loss & mass Rt side neck & foreign body sensation throat x 4m	fungating growth Rt vallecula & epiglottis	malignant	supraglottic
24	mass Lt side neck x 6m, pain Lt ear x 1yr	growth Lt vallecula & epiglottis	malignant	supraglottic
25	weight loss x 3m	ulcerative growth Rt false vocal cord & Rt arytenoid	malignant	supraglottic
26	-	exophytic growth involving all of epiglottis	malignant	supraglottic
27	appetite & weight loss x 20 days	exophytic growth Lt false vocal cord & Lt arytenoid	malignant	supraglottic
28	haemoptysis & pain throat x 2m, weight loss x 3m	exophytic growth Rt aryepiglottic fold	malignant	supraglottic

29	-	small growth Rt vocal cord	benign	glottic
30	cough & sore throat x 6m	smooth mass Rt aryepiglottic fold & Rt pyriform fossa	malignant	supraglottic
31	-	fungating growth Rt vocal cord extending to subglottis	malignant	glottic & subglottic
32	cough & sore throat x 1m	reddish globular growth Rt vocal cord	malignant	glottic
33	appetite & weight loss x 6m, haemoptysis x 15d	extensive growth Lt epiglottis & pyriform fossa	malignant	supraglottic
34	haemoptysis x 15d	fungating growth Rt aryepiglottic fold & pyriform fossa	malignant	supraglottic
35	cough & sore throat x 20d	growth involving Rt arytenoid & Rt aryepiglottic fold	benign	supraglottic
36	cough & sore throat & haemoptysis x 1m	growth involving Rt aryepiglottic fold & Rt vocal cord	malignant	supraglottic & glottic
37	fever & haemoptysis x 3m	growth involving Lt false and true vocal cords	malignant	supraglottic & glottic
38	cough & sore throat	bilateral vocal cord polyps	benign	glottic

	x 2yr, foreign body sensation throat x 1y			
39	-	bilateral vocal nodules	benign	glottic
40	cough & sore throat x 3m	bilateral vocal nodules	benign	glottic
41	-	growth Lt vocal cord	benign	glottic
42	foreign body sensation throat x 3m	polyp Rt vocal cord	benign	glottic
43	-	Rt vocal nodule	benign	glottic
44	-	small growth Rt vocal cord	malignant	glottic
45	haemoptysis x 1m	polypoidal mass Lt vocal cord	benign	glottic
46	cough & sore throat x 8m	ulcerating growth Rt vocal cord	malignant	glottic
47	appetite & weight loss x 6m	fungating growth epiglottis	malignant	supraglottic
48	foreign body sensation throat x 1yr	cystic growth Rt vocal cord	malignant	glottic
49	-	globular mass on Rt vocal cord	benign	glottic

| 50 | - | ulcerative growth on tip of epiglottis | malignant | supraglottic |

MASTER CHART contd. Lab Investigations

SN	Lab Investigations (Hb %)	Histopathological diagnosis	Tracheostomy done Yes/No
1	12gm%	well differentiated Sq Cell Ca	Yes
2	10.8gm%	inflammatory nodules	No
3	11gm%	well differentiated Sq Cell Ca	No
4	13.5gm%	stratified Sq epithelium with small cysts	No
5	12gm%	papillary Sq Cell Ca	Yes
6	11gm%	epidermoid carcinoma in situ	No
7	11gm%	stratified Sq lining with parakeratosis subepi oedematous	No
8	13.5gm%	Sq epithelium with hyperplasia	No
9	12gm%	Sq epi with papillomatous hyperplasia	No
10	12.5gm%	Sq epi with salivary glands	No
11	11.2gm%	well differentiated Sq Cell Ca	No
12	13.5gm%	papillary Sq Cell Ca	No
13	11gm%	Sq Cell Papilloma	No
14	12gm%	Sq epi with mild dysplasia & congested blood vessels	No
15	13gm%	well differentiated Sq Cell Ca	No

16	13gm%	well differentiated Sq Cell Ca	Yes
17	9.5gm%	moderately differentiated Sq Cell Ca	No
18	14gm%	well differentiated Sq Cell Ca	No
19	10.5gm%	stratified Sq epi & subepi congested	No
20	12gm%	Sq epi with parakeratosis & subepi congested	No
21	12gm%	poorly differentiated Sq Cell Ca	No
22	10.2gm%	well differentiated Sq Cell Ca	No
23	12gm%	moderately differentiated Sq Cell Ca	No
24	10gm%	well differentiated Sq Cell Ca	No
25	10.5gm%	well differentiated Sq Cell Ca	Yes
26	10gm%	poorly differentiated Sq Cell Ca	Yes
27	12gm%	moderately differentiated Sq Cell Ca	Yes
28	10gm%	well differentiated Sq Cell Ca	No
29	10gm%	Sq epi with hyperplasia	No
30	13gm%	moderately differentiated Sq Cell Ca	Yes
31	12.4gm%	well differentiated Sq Cell Ca	No
32	10.5gm%	moderately differentiated Sq Cell Ca	No
33	10.5gm%	moderately differentiated Sq Cell Ca	Yes
34	13gm%	poorly differentiated Sq Cell Ca	No
35	12gm%	Sq epi with papillomatous hyperplasia	Yes
36	12.5gm%	basaloid Sq Cell Ca	No
37	11.2gm%	well differentiated Sq Cell Ca	Yes

38	14.6gm%	stratified Sq epi & subepi showing amorphous material	No
39	12gm%	stratified Sq epi with hyperplasia	No
40	13gm%	Sq epi & subepi oedematous	No
41	12.8gm%	Sq epi with papillomatous hyperplasia	No
42	11gm%	Sq epi with subepi showing inflammatory cells	No
43	10.2gm%	Sq epi with parakeratosis & subepi congested	No
44	10gm%	moderately differentiated Sq Cell Ca	No
45	13.6gm%	Sq epi with parakeratosis	No
46	13gm%	well differentiated Sq Cell Ca	No
47	12gm%	well differentiated Sq Cell Ca	No
48	8gm%	moderately differentiated Sq Cell Ca	No
49	12gm%	stratified Sq epi with hyperplasia & subepi showing myxoid changes	No
50	12.6gm%	well differentiated Sq Cell Ca	No

Abbreviations used in Master Chart:
Lt - Left;
Rt - Right;
Sq - Squamous;
epi - epithelium;
subepi - subepithelium;
Ca - Carcinoma;

d - days; m - months; yr - years; M - Male; F – Female

INDEX

A

B

D

E

55, 59, 68-80, 82-5, 87-89,
91-2, 94-9, 101-3
benign growth(s), 49, 79, 89, 98
benign epithelial neoplasm, 98
bilateral polyps, 11
biopsy, 17, 20, 50, 52-3, 56-7, 65,
67, 90, 102, 116

C

Cancer, laryngeal 15-17, 20, 49,
93-7, 100, 105-7
larynx 20, 47, 51, 53-4,
58, 90, 92-7, 105, 108,
110
carcinoid tumour(s), 18, 50, 53
carcinoma of larynx   18, 47, 54,
60, 92, 94-5, 97-8, 111
cartilages, 25-6
arytenoid 19, 22, 25-31, 33,
116, 124-6
corniculate 25, 27-8, 43
cricoid 14, 24-9, 30-3, 42, 50-1,
55
cuneiform 25, 27, 30, 43

H

Haemangioma(s), 13, 49
hoarseness, 16, 53-5, 59, 80-2,
97-8, 103, 113, 120
human papilloma virus, 15
HPV6, 59
HPV11, 12, 59, 96
hyalinization, 11, 99
haemoptysis, 54, 82-3, 97-8, 103,
125-6
hyperplasia,   13, 17, 84-85, 87,
127, 129-30

6
histopathological 20, 57, 65,
90, 102
ENT 67
extrinsic ligaments,
membranes, muscle 25, 28-9,
33, 59, 106

F

False vocal cord, false cord 14, 22, 30,
41, 44, 52,
116, 123-6
fibromas, 14
fibrous polyps, 11
fine needle aspiration, FNA 17
fortwin, injection 65

G

Glottis, 10, 22-3, 31, 56
granular cell, tumours, myoblastomas,
14, 49

ligament,
cricotracheal 28-9
cricothyroid 26, 28-30, 33, 35,
37
Hyoepiglottic, 28-9
Thyroepiglottic, 27-9
Lipoma(s), lipomatous 14, 49-52, 56,
91, 105, 112
Liposarcoma(s), 19, 51, 112
lymphangiomas, 13
lymphatic drainage, lymphatics, 37-8
lymphoepithelioma,
lymphoepitheliomatous 17-8
lymphoma(s), 17, 19, 48, 54, 56, 104,
106

About the Author

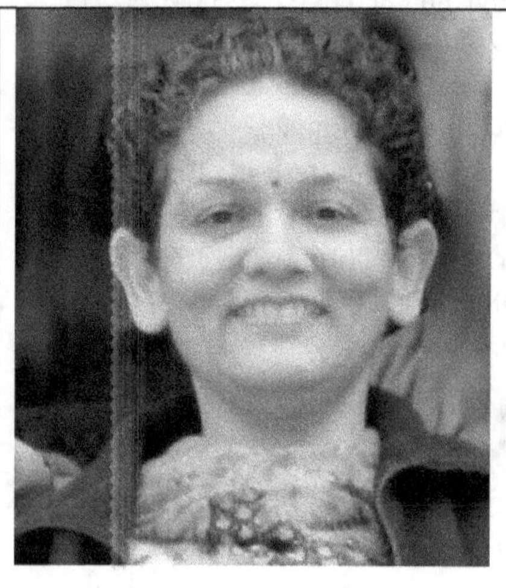

Dr Sangeeta Aggarwal is with Rajendra Medical College and Hospital, Patiala as Senior Resident in the department of ENT.

She is an avid home maker and a medical professional with a penchant for attending devotional satsangs. She loves cooking and organizing Art of Living courses.

Editor

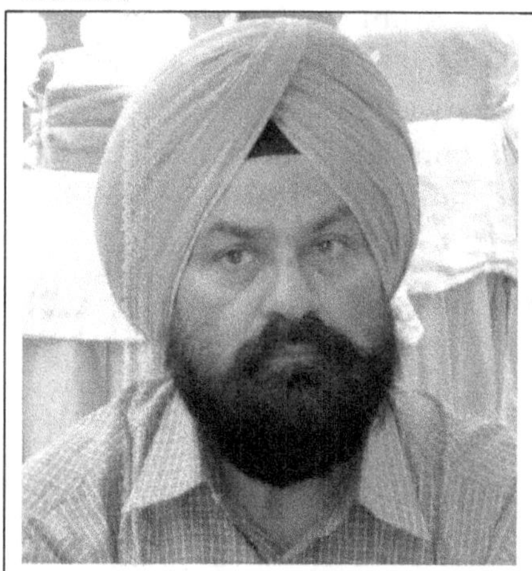

Dr Barjinder Singh Sohal is Associate Professor with the ENT department of GMCH, Patiala. He has a rich teaching experience of 16 years, and has published 7 papers in reputed medical journals.

He takes utmost interest in the professional growth of his medical staff, and strives for complete treatment and ethical care of his patients. Loves to organize medical camps for the rural population. An avid hockey player and encourages extracurricular activities in the college.

Published Papers

Suicidal Cut Throat Injury And Successful Repair

JEMDS (Journal of Evolution of Medical and Dental Sciences)
Year: 2019, Month: February, Volume: 8, Issue: 8, Page: 544-546

https://www.jemds.com/latest-articles.php?at_id=16655

Tonsillolith As A Cause Of Glossopharyngeal Neuralgia- An Unusual Entity

JEMDS (Journal of Evolution of Medical and Dental Sciences)
Year: 2018, Month: November, Volume: 7, Issue:46, Page: 5055-5056

https://www.jemds.com/data_pdf/1_sangeeta%20aggarwal--Nov-12-CR.pdf

Isolated Sphenoid Pyocele with Thornwaldt's Cyst of Nasopharynx

IJOHNS (Indian Journal of Otolaryngology and Head and Neck Surgery
Year: 2011, Month: July, Volume: 63, Supplement: 1, Page: 140-141

https://pubmed.ncbi.nlm.nih.gov/22754866/

Epilogue

सर्वे भवन्तु सुखिनः । सर्वे सन्तु निरामयाः ।

सर्वे भद्राणि पश्यन्तु । मा कश्चिद् दुःख भाग् भवेत् ॥

ॐ शान्तिः शान्तिः शान्तिः ॥

sarve bhavantu sukhinaḥ | sarve santu nirāmayāḥ |

sarve bhadrāṇi paśyantu | mā kaścid duḥkha bhāg bhavet ||

oṃ śāntiḥ śāntiḥ śāntiḥ ||

May all be BLISSFUL. May all be HEALTHY.
May all see the AUSPICIOUS in Man & Nature. May
none go astray nor be prey to wickedness.

When faith has blossomed in life, Every step is led by the Divine.

Sri Sri Ravi Shankar

Om Namah Shivaya

जय गुरुदेव